Peate's Body Systems

Peate's Body Systems

The Eyes

Ian Peate, OBE FRCN EN(G) RGN DipN(Lond) RNT BEd(Hons) MA(Lond) LLM

Editor in Chief, British Journal of Nursing;
Consultant Editor, Journal of Paramedic Practice;
Consultant Editor, International Journal for Advancing Practice;
Visiting Professor, Northumbria University;
Visiting Professor, Buckinghamshire New University;
Professorial Fellow, University of Roehampton;
Visiting Senior Clinical Fellow, University of Hertfordshire

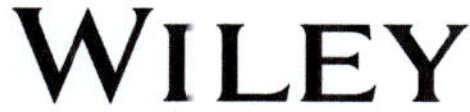

Contents

Preface ix

Acknowledgements xi

1 Anatomy and Physiology: The Eyes 1

The Sense of Sight 1

The Anatomy and Physiology of the Eye 4

Conjunctiva 6

Lacrimal Apparatus 7

The Eye 8

Organisation of the Retina 10

Colour Vision and Retinal Structure 10

Eye Chambers 12

Focusing Images on the Retina 12

Refraction 12

Focal Length 13

Myopia, Hyperopia and Presbyopia 14

Processing of Visual Information 15

Central Processing of Visual Information 15

Conclusion 16

Glossary of Terms 16

Multiple Choice Questions 17

References 19

2 Assessment of the Eyes 20

Importance of Vision Assessment 20

The Assessment 21

Patient History in Ophthalmic Assessment 24

Documentation of Findings 24

Testing Visual Function 27

LogMAR Vision Testing 29

Tumbling 'E', 'E' Test 29

Colour Vision Assessment 30

Diagnostic Tests 31

Conclusion 33

Glossary of Terms 34

Multiple Choice Questions 35

References 36

3 Glaucoma 37

Pathophysiological Changes Associated with Primary Open-angle Glaucoma 37

Epidemiology 39

Risk Factors 41

Clinical Presentation 42

Clinical Investigations and Diagnosis 43

Management 44

Health Teaching 47

Conclusion 49

Glossary of Terms 50

Multiple Choice Questions 51

References 52

4 Cataract 54

Pathophysiological Changes Associated with Cataract 56

Epidemiology 58

Risk Factors 59

Clinical Presentation 59

Clinical Investigations and Diagnosis 61

Management 64

Surgical Management 65

Cataract Surgery Procedure 65

Types of Intra-optical Lenses 66

Postoperative Care 66

Health Teaching 66

Conclusion 69

Glossary of Terms 70

Multiple Choice Questions 71

References 72

5 Conjunctivitis 73

Pink Eye 73

Viral Conjunctivitis 73

Bacterial Conjunctivitis 73

Allergic Conjunctivitis 73

Chemical Conjunctivitis 73

Giant Papillary Conjunctivitis 74

Neonatal Conjunctivitis 74

Non-infectious Conjunctivitis 74

Pathophysiological Changes Associated with Conjunctivitis 74

Conjunctival Anatomy and Function 75

Types of Conjunctivitis and Specific Pathophysiological Mechanisms 76

Protective Mechanisms and Self-limiting Nature 77

Epidemiology 78

Ophthalmia Neonatorum 78

Risk Factors 79

General Risks Across All Types 80

Populations at Higher Risk 80

Clinical Presentation 81

Clinical Investigations and Diagnosis 83

Management 87

Bacterial Conjunctivitis 87

Viral Conjunctivitis 88

Allergic Conjunctivitis 88

Chemical Conjunctivitis 88

Further Considerations 89

Health Teaching 89

Conclusion 90

Glossary of Terms 91

Multiple Choice Questions 92

References 93

6 Age-related Macular Degeneration 94

Macular Degeneration 94

Pathophysiological Changes Associated with Age-related Macular Degeneration 95

Dry (Non-exudative or Atrophic) 95

Wet (Neovascular or Exudative) Age-related Macular Degeneration 97

Epidemiology 99

Risk Factors 99

Clinical Presentation 100

Dry Age-related Macular
Degeneration (Atrophic)   101

Wet Age-related Macular
Degeneration (Neovascular
or Exudative)   101

General Symptoms of Age-related
Macular Degeneration   102

Clinical Investigations
and Diagnosis   103

Initial Consultation   103

Symptom Inquiry   104

Structured Interviews and
Questionnaires   104

Documentation and
Follow-up   105

Visual Acuity Test   106

Amsler Grid Test   106

Fundoscopic Examination
(Ophthalmoscopy)   106

Optical Coherence
Tomography   106

Fluorescein Angiography   107

Indocyanine Green
Angiography   107

Fundus Autofluorescence   107

Electroretinography   107

Management   107

Health Teaching   109

Conclusion   110

Glossary of Terms   111

Multiple Choice Questions   112

References   113

7   Retinitis   114

Retinal Dystrophies   114

Types   114

Symptoms   115

Causes   115

Pathophysiological Changes
Associated with Retinitis
Pigmentosa   116

Genetic Mutations   116

Photoreceptor Degeneration   116

Retinal Pigment Epithelium
Changes   117

Vascular Changes   117

Retinal Remodelling   117

Inflammatory Responses   117

Secondary Effects   117

Clinical Implications   117

Epidemiology   118

Risk Factors   118

Genetic Mutations   118

Environmental and Lifestyle
Factors   119

Age of Onset   120

Clinical Presentation   120

Initial Symptoms   120

Clinical Investigations and
Diagnosis   122

Patient History   122

Symptom Onset and
Progression   122

Central Vision Changes   123

Family History   123

Previous Ocular and Medical
History   123

Visual Function Impact   124

Psychosocial Aspects   124

Examination and
Investigations   125

Clinical Examination   125

Retinal Imaging   125

Functional Tests   126

Genetic Testing   126

Additional Tests   126

Visual Field Testing
(Perimetry) 127

Management 127

Gene Therapy 128

Health Teaching 129

Conclusion 130

Glossary of Terms 130

Multiple Choice Questions 131

References 132

8 Presbyopia **134**

Myopia, Hyperopia and
Presbyopia 134

Emmetropia 134

Refractive Error 134

Pathophysiological Changes
Associated with Presbyopia 134

Epidemiology 137

Risk Factors 138

Clinical Presentation 140

Clinical Investigations and
Diagnosis 140

Management 143

Health Teaching 143

Conclusion 145

Glossary of Terms 146

Multiple Choice Questions 147

References 148

MCQ Answers **150**

Index **151**

Preface

Welcome to *Peate's Body Systems*; there are 12 books in the series. This is a comprehensive collection of textbooks designed to support and enrich the knowledge of health and care workers across various fields. This series is intended to be a valuable resource for those who are dedicated to understanding the intricacies of human biology, physiology and the various systems that sustain life.

Peate's Body Systems series is rooted in the belief that a deep and thorough understanding of the human body is essential for providing the highest standard of care. Each book in this series is thoroughly crafted to offer clear, accurate and up-to-date information on different body systems. The aim is to bridge the gap between complex scientific concepts and practical, everyday applications in healthcare settings.

PURPOSE AND SCOPE

The purpose of this series is to provide health and care workers with:

- Foundational knowledge, with explanations of the anatomical structures and physiological functions of the body systems

- Insights into how these systems interact with each other and how they are impacted by various diseases and conditions, highlighting clinical relevance and encouraging practical application

STRUCTURE OF THE SERIES

Each book in *Peate's Body Systems* focuses on a specific body system:

The Cardiovascular System	The Female Reproductive System
The Respiratory System	The Male Reproductive System
The Digestive System	The Musculoskeletal System
The Renal System	The Skin
The Nervous System	The Ear, Nose and Throat
The Endocrine System	The Eyes

Every chapter is designed to be comprehensive yet accessible, making complex information easier to digest and apply. Figures, tables, boxes, illustrations and flowcharts have been extensively used to support visual learning and reinforce key concepts.

This series is tailored for:

- Healthcare students: those in nursing and allied health programmes

- Practicing professionals: nurses, therapists and other care workers seeking to deepen their understanding and stay current with the latest developments in health and care

- Educators and trainers: educators who require reliable and comprehensive teaching materials to advise and instruct the next generation of healthcare providers

Commitment to Excellence. The series is committed to providing quality educational resources that not only inform but also inspire and empower health and care workers. By equipping you with a robust understanding of the systems of life, you will be better prepared to make informed decisions, deliver compassionate care and ultimately improve patient outcomes.

Thank you for choosing *Peate's Body Systems* as your trusted resource. I hope these textbooks serve as a valuable tool in your ongoing journey of learning and professional development.

IAN PEATE
London

Acknowledgements

I would like to acknowledge the help and support of my partner Jussi Lahtinen. Acknowledgements also go to staff at the RCN Library in London. My thanks go to Tom Marriott, Christabel Daniel Raj, Bhavya Boopathi and all those at Wiley.

Anatomy and Physiology: The Eyes

CHAPTER 1

THE SENSE OF SIGHT

The sense of sight holds immense importance due to its multifaceted role in human life. It spans biological, psychological and social dimensions.

From a biological perspective, sight is essential for survival. It allows individuals to detect potential dangers in their environment, such as predators or hazardous conditions, enhancing their ability to avoid threats. Additionally, vision facilitates precise navigation and spatial orientation, enabling effective movement and coordination in complex surroundings.

In terms of information processing, vision provides access to complex visual data, including a wide range of colours, shapes and movements. This detailed information is vital for making informed decisions. The human visual system processes this data with remarkable speed and efficiency, which is particularly critical in scenarios that require quick responses, such as driving or playing sports.

Socially, sight plays a pivotal role in communication and interaction. A significant portion of human communication is non-verbal, relying on visual cues such as facial expressions, gestures and body language. These visual signals are essential for understanding and responding to others, thereby fostering social bonds and enhancing empathy. Eye contact and visual recognition are also key elements in forming and maintaining relationships within a community.

Sight is integral to learning and development. Visual aids such as books, diagrams and digital media are fundamental in educational settings, helping individuals to comprehend and retain information. Additionally, many skills are acquired and refined through visual observation and imitation, highlighting the importance of sight in personal and professional growth.

The artistic and cultural appreciation enabled by vision enriches human experience. The ability to see allows individuals to enjoy the beauty of art, nature and architecture, contributing to cultural and personal enrichment. Furthermore, visual perception stimulates creativity and innovation, impacting fields such as design, technology and the arts.

Economically and practically, vision is vital across numerous professions. Many jobs, from healthcare to engineering, depend heavily on visual skills for accuracy and efficiency. Visual inspections are crucial in various industries to ensure quality control and safety, directly influencing productivity and reducing risks.

The sense of sight is integral to human functioning and well-being. It enhances interaction with the environment, supports cognitive and social development and contributes to cultural and aesthetic experiences. The myriad ways in which sight underpins daily activities, professional tasks and overall quality of life underscore its profound importance and should not be underestimated. Table 1.1 provides an overview of the sense of sight.

When vision fails or deteriorates, it significantly impacts various aspects of life, ranging from practical day-to-day activities to broader social and psychological well-being, and it can lead to a significant loss of independence. Navigating environments becomes difficult and often unsafe, resulting in increased dependence on others for transportation and movement.

Table 1.1   The sense of sight

Biological function and survival	Detection of danger: Vision allows for the detection of potential threats in the environment, such as predators, hazardous terrain or other dangers, enhancing survival.
	Navigation and coordination: Sight enables precise navigation and spatial orientation; this facilitates movement and coordination in complex environments.
Information processing	Complex visual data: The human eye can perceive a vast range of colours, shapes and movements, providing detailed information about the surroundings. This data is key for making informed decisions.
	Speed and efficiency: Visual processing is highly efficient, allowing for the rapid interpretation of vast amounts of information. This efficiency is critical in tasks requiring quick responses, such as driving or sports.
Communication and social interaction	Non-verbal cues: A significant portion of human communication is non-verbal, relying on facial expressions, gestures and body language, all of which are then interpreted visually.
	Social bonding: Eye contact and visual recognition play important roles in forming and maintaining social bonds, enhancing empathy and fostering community.
Learning and development	Educational tools: Visual aids such as books, diagrams and digital media are essential tools in education, facilitating learning and comprehension.
	Skill acquisition: Many skills, from basic tasks to complex procedures, are learned and then refined through visual observation and imitation.
	Aesthetic and cultural appreciation:
	Art and nature: Sight allows individuals to appreciate the beauty of art, nature and architecture. This can enrich cultural and personal experiences.
	Creativity and innovation: Visual perception stimulates creativity and innovation, influencing fields such as design, technology and the arts.
Economic and practical implications	Occupational roles: Numerous professions, from healthcare to engineering, depend heavily on visual skills for accuracy and efficiency.
	Productivity and safety: In many industries, visual inspections ensure quality control and safety, impacting productivity and reducing risks.

Daily activities that rely heavily on sight, such as reading, cooking and personal grooming, may become challenging, diminishing a person's ability to perform these tasks independently.

Health and safety risks are also heightened with vision impairment. Poor vision increases the risk of falls, collisions and other accidents, both at home and in public spaces. Additionally, vision impairments can delay the detection of other health issues that have visible symptoms, complicating overall healthcare and leading to potentially severe consequences if not addressed promptly.

Visual impairment can contribute to cognitive decline, as it limits engagement in stimulating activities that are essential for maintaining cognitive function. Furthermore, vision loss can lead to depression, anxiety and social isolation due to the challenges and frustrations associated with decreased independence and reduced ability to engage in previously enjoyed activities.

Social implications are significant as well. Individuals with vision loss might withdraw from social activities due to embarrassment or logistical difficulties; this can lead to feelings of loneliness and isolation.

The economic and occupational impacts are considerable. Many jobs require good vision, and deterioration in eyesight can limit job opportunities or necessitate early retirement. Moreover, the financial burden associated with the cost of assistive devices, medical treatments and necessary home modifications can be substantial, placing a strain on individuals and families.

Educational barriers are another critical issue. For both children and adults, vision loss can thwart the ability to read, write and engage with educational materials, potentially impacting academic performance and lifelong learning.

Vision loss significantly affects the quality of life. Activities such as watching television, reading and enjoying nature become less accessible, diminishing overall enjoyment. While assistive technologies can help mitigate some challenges, they may not fully compensate for the loss of natural vision and can be expensive or difficult to use.

The deterioration or loss of vision has profound and far-reaching effects. It compromises independence, heightens health and safety risks, affects mental and emotional well-being and imposes significant social, economic and educational challenges (Clare 2020). Addressing these impacts requires a combination of medical intervention, assistive technologies and support systems to help individuals adapt and maintain their quality of life.

Those who offer care and support to people with a visual disturbance have a key role to play in helping to address the challenges that arise from vision loss or deterioration. To effectively manage these issues, a comprehensive approach involving prevention, early detection, treatment, rehabilitation and support services is essential.

Prevention and early detection are important steps. Regular eye examinations are vital for detecting vision issues early, especially in high-risk groups such as the elderly, those with diabetes and those with a family history of eye diseases. Public health education is equally important, as it informs people about the significance of eye health, the risks associated with vision loss and the benefits of protective measures such as wearing sunglasses, managing chronic conditions and avoiding smoking.

When it comes to medical and surgical interventions, those offering care and support should discuss appropriate treatments for conditions such as glaucoma, macular degeneration and diabetic retinopathy to slow their progression and manage symptoms. Surgical solutions, such as cataract surgery, can often restore vision and significantly improve the patients' quality of life.

Addressing the psychological impact of vision loss is also essential. Counselling services can help patients cope with the emotional and psychological challenges, while support groups offer a sense of community and shared experience. Integrated mental health services can address issues including depression and anxiety, ensuring comprehensive care for patients.

Social and educational support systems are necessary to help individuals adapt to their vision loss. Social services can assist with mobility training, access to transportation and home adaptations.

Technological aids such as screen readers, text-to-speech software and smartphone apps that have been designed for the visually impaired are invaluable. Providing training on these tools is essential for effective use. Adaptive devices such as white canes, guide dogs and specialised GPS systems also help improve mobility and independence.

A comprehensive care coordination approach is essential, involving an interdisciplinary team of ophthalmologists, optometrists, care workers, primary care physicians, occupational therapists, psychologists and social workers. This team can address the multifaceted needs of patients with vision loss. Developing patient-centred care plans, with the patient at the heart of all that is done, ensures that care is tailored to each individual's specific needs, preferences and goals.

Those who offer care and support to people can advocate for better public transportation options, workplace accommodation and policies that support individuals.

Adopting these strategies can help to mitigate the impact of vision loss and help patients lead fuller, more independent lives.

The special senses are smell, taste, vision and hearing (these include equilibrium). They are known as the special senses because their sensory receptors are located within relatively large sensory organs located in the head – the nose, tongue, eyes and ears. The skin is sometimes considered a sense organ.

THE ANATOMY AND PHYSIOLOGY OF THE EYE

The eyes and their associated structures are intricate sensory organs that facilitate vision. When there are no visual impairments, light rays are refracted as they pass through the different layers of the tear film, cornea, pupil, lens, vitreous humour and finally reach the macula on the retina. At this point, the light is converted into nerve impulses that travel through the optic nerve to the occipital lobe in the brain, where images are processed and recognised (Sanderson 2019). Eye examinations can reveal many systemic health issues.

The sense of sight is based on the eyes and around the eyes, there are a number of accessory structures that help to keep the eyes safe and working well (see Figure 1.1).

Eyebrows: Eyebrows serve several important functions related to the protection and expression of the eyes:

- Shade and sun protection: Help to shield the eyes from direct sunlight. By reducing the amount of light that reaches the eyes, they contribute to better vision in bright conditions and help to prevent glare, which can be uncomfortable and potentially harmful over prolonged periods.

- Barrier against moisture and debris: Eyebrows are effective in diverting sweat, rain and other moisture away from the eyes. Their arching shape directs these liquids to the sides of

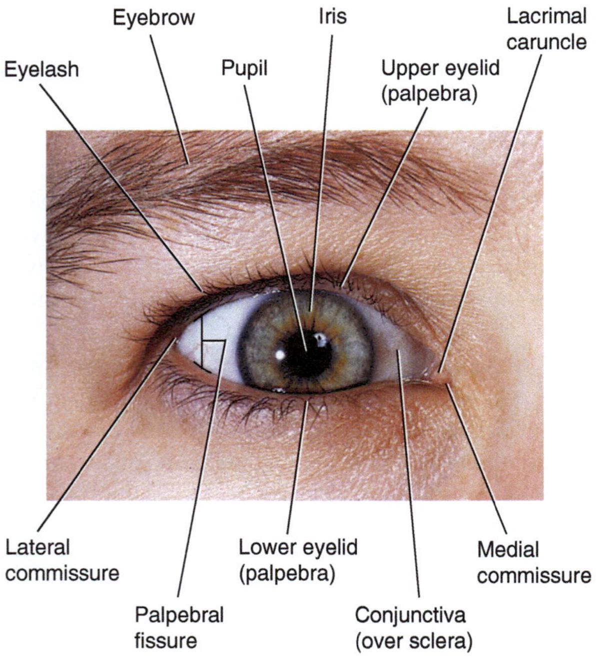

FIGURE 1.1 Accessory structures of the eye

the face, preventing them from running directly into the eyes. This helps maintain clear vision and protects the delicate eye surface from potential irritation and contamination by salts and other substances found in sweat.

- Debris protection: The thick hairs of the eyebrows also act as a physical barrier, catching and trapping dust, dirt and other small particles that might otherwise fall into the eyes. This function is important in environments with a lot of airborne debris.

- Expression and communication: Beyond their protective roles, eyebrows play a significant part in non-verbal communication. Movements and positions of the eyebrows can convey a wide range of emotions, including surprise, anger, joy and concern. This aspect of eyebrows is important for social interactions, helping to express feelings and intentions clearly to others.

- Aesthetic and identity: Eyebrows contribute to the aesthetic aspect of the face and are a key component of individual identity. Their shape, thickness and colour can significantly affect one's appearance. Grooming and styling eyebrows have become important aspects for some people with regard to personal care and fashion, highlighting their role in facial aesthetics.

Eyebrows are multifunctional features that provide essential protection against environmental elements, contribute to facial expression and enhance personal identity and aesthetics.

Eyelids (also called palpebrae): They are extensions of the skin that continuously blink to lubricate the eye's surface and remove debris. The space located between the eyelids is called the palpebral fissure.

Eyelashes: The eyelashes are strong hairs that protect the eyes from foreign particles. They are linked to the tarsal glands; these glands produce a lipid-rich secretion that prevents the eyelids from sticking together.

Lacrimal caruncle: This is a small, fleshy bump that is situated at the inner corner of the eye, near the medial canthus (the point where the upper and lower eyelids meet closest to the nose). This structure is composed of soft tissue and includes a variety of accessory glands, such as sebaceous glands, sweat glands and sometimes even a few lacrimal (tear) glands.

These glands play a crucial role in maintaining the health and function of the eye. The sebaceous glands produce an oily substance that helps to lubricate the eye and prevent the tear film from evaporating too quickly. The sweat glands contribute to the moisture of the ocular surface. In some cases, the lacrimal glands present in the lacrimal caruncle also contribute to tear production, which is essential for keeping the eye surface moist and free from dust and other irritants.

Commissure: The term commissure in the anatomical context refers to the points where structures come together or join. In the case of the eyelids, the commissures are the areas where the upper and lower eyelids meet. These are essential landmarks for both functional and aesthetic considerations in ophthalmology and plastic surgery. There are two types of commissures.

LATERAL COMMISSURE (CANTHUS)

- Location: This is the outer corner of the eye, where the upper and lower eyelids meet closest to the temple.

- Function: The lateral commissure plays a role in the lateral extension of the eyelids and contributes to the overall shape and opening of the eye. It is also involved in the drainage of tears through the lacrimal system.

- Anatomical structures: Nearby structures include the lateral palpebral ligament, which helps in maintaining the position and stability of the lateral commissure.

MEDIAL COMMISSURE (CANTHUS)

- Location: This is the inner corner of the eye, where the upper and lower eyelids meet closest to the nose.

- Function: The medial commissure is crucial for the drainage of tears. It contains the lacrimal caruncle and the plica semilunaris (a small fold of conjunctiva). The tear drainage system, including the puncta (small openings on the eyelid margins that lead to the lacrimal sac), is located near this commissure.

- Anatomical structures: It includes the medial palpebral ligament and lacrimal apparatus components such as the lacrimal sac and nasolacrimal duct, which are essential for tear drainage into the nasal cavity.

Understanding the commissures' anatomy is vital for diagnosing and treating various ocular and periocular conditions (it has clinical significance):

- Infections and inflammation: Conditions such as blepharitis (inflammation of the eyelids) or dacryocystitis (infection of the lacrimal sac) often involve the medial commissure.

- Trauma and surgery: Knowledge of the commissural anatomy is crucial during reconstructive surgery, eyelid laceration repairs and cosmetic procedures such as blepharoplasty.

- Tear drainage disorders: Blockage or dysfunction in the tear drainage system, often linked to the medial commissure, can lead to conditions that include epiphora (excessive tearing).

CONJUNCTIVA

A thin, transparent mucous membrane composed of epithelial cells. It serves a critical role in protecting and maintaining the health of the eye. This membrane is divided into two main parts:

- Palpebral conjunctiva: This section lines the inside surface of the eyelids, creating a protective barrier between the delicate inner tissues of the eyelid and the external environment. It helps to keep the inner eyelid smooth and moist, ensuring comfortable movement of the eyelids over the eye's surface.

- Bulbar conjunctiva: This portion covers the anterior part of the sclera (the white part of the eye), extending from the edge of the cornea to the area just beyond the visible part of the sclera. Although it is transparent, it is rich in blood vessels, which can sometimes become visible when the eye is irritated or inflamed.

The conjunctiva has several important functions:

- It acts as a protective barrier for the eye, protecting it from dust, debris and microorganisms. The conjunctiva's immune components help to prevent infections.

- The conjunctiva produces mucus and tears that contribute to the tear film, which keeps the eye surface moist and lubricated, facilitating smooth movement of the eyelids and reducing friction.

- It plays a role in the healing process of the eye by producing enzymes and growth factors that aid in tissue repair.

Overall, the conjunctiva is essential for maintaining the eye's health and functionality, contributing to both its defence mechanisms and its smooth operation.

LACRIMAL APPARATUS

The lacrimal apparatus ensures a constant flow of tears over the eyes; the aim is to keep the conjunctiva moist and clean. Tears serve several important functions:

- Reduce friction

- Remove debris

- Prevent bacterial infection

- Provide nutrients and oxygen to parts of the conjunctiva

The lacrimal apparatus is responsible for producing, distributing and removing tears. It consists of:

- Lacrimal gland

- Lacrimal canaliculi

- Lacrimal sac

- Nasolacrimal duct

The lacrimal gland (tear gland) produces most of the tear content, about 1 mL per day (Clare 2020), (see Figure 1.2). Once the lacrimal secretions reach the eye, they mix with products from the accessory and tarsal glands; this creates a mixture that lubricates the eye and reduces evaporation. The corneal cells' nutrient and oxygen needs are met by diffusion from

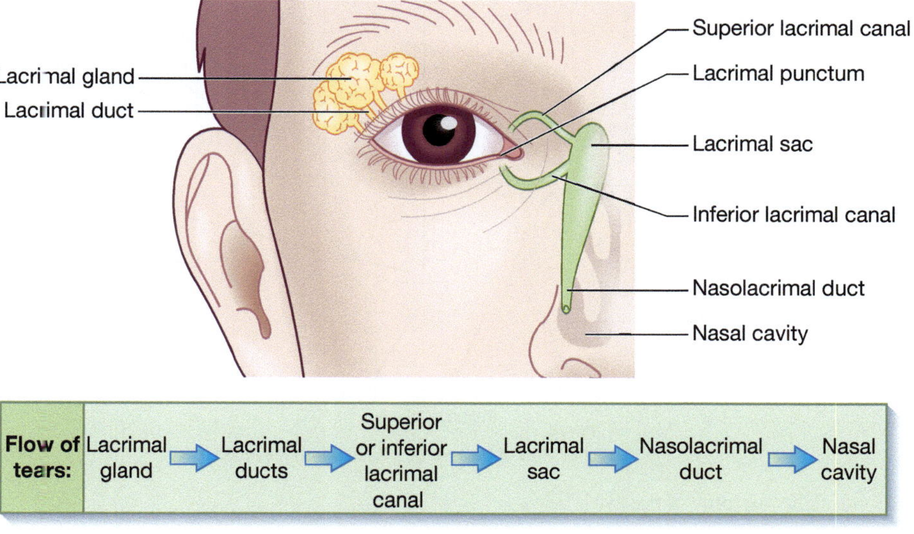

FIGURE 1.2   The lacrimal apparatus

these secretions. Additionally, the secretions contain antibacterial enzymes and antibodies to combat pathogens before they enter the body.

Blinking sweeps tears across the ocular surface, accumulating at the medial commissure. From there, they are drained by the lacrimal canaliculi into the lacrimal sac and then into the nasal cavity through the nasolacrimal duct.

THE EYE

The eye, a globe, has three layers (Figure 1.3):

1. Fibrous tunic

2. Vascular tunic

3. Neural tunic

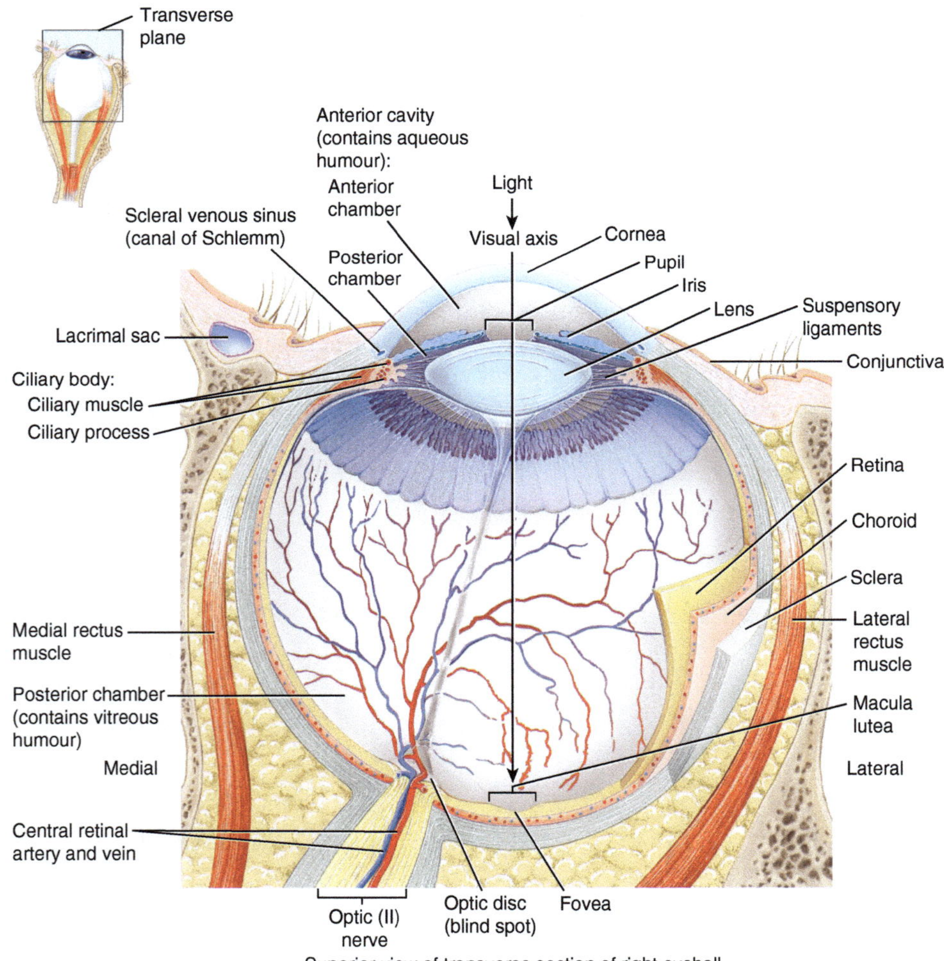

FIGURE 1.3 The anatomy of the eye

THE FIBROUS TUNIC

The fibrous tunic is the outermost layer of the eye, comprising the sclera and cornea. It has three main functions; it provides support and protection, serves as the attachment site for extrinsic muscles and contains structures that aid in the focusing process.

The majority of the ocular surface is covered by the sclera, known as the 'white' of the eye. The sclera consists of dense fibrous connective tissue with collagen and elastic fibres. Its surface contains small blood vessels and nerves. The transparent cornea is continuous with the sclera and consists of a dense matrix of fibres that are arranged to allow the passage of light without interference.

VASCULAR TUNIC (UVEA)

The vascular tunic is the middle layer of the eye, containing numerous blood vessels, lymph vessels and smooth muscles essential for eye function. Its functions include:

- Providing a structure for blood and lymph vessels that supply the eye tissues

- Regulating the amount of light entering the eye

- Secreting and reabsorbing aqueous humour

- Controlling the shape of the lens

The vascular tunic is composed of three parts:

- Iris

- Ciliary body

- Choroid

Iris   The iris is the central, coloured part of the eye that regulates light entry by adjusting the size of the pupil. It consists of two layers of pigmented cells, fibres and two layers of smooth muscle (pupillary muscles):

- Pupillary constrictor muscles

- Pupillary dilator muscles

These muscles are controlled by the autonomic nervous system. The parasympathetic nervous system causes pupil constriction in response to bright light, while the sympathetic nervous system causes pupil dilation in dim light. The edge of the iris attaches to the anterior part of the ciliary body.

Ciliary Body   The ciliary body primarily consists of the ciliary muscle, a smooth muscular ring that projects into the eye's interior. Its epithelial covering has many folds that are called ciliary processes, to which the suspensory ligaments of the lens attach.

Choroid   The choroid is a vascular layer that separates the fibrous and neural tunics. It lies beneath the sclera and is attached to the outermost layer of the retina. The choroid contains a vast capillary network that supplies oxygen and nutrients to the retina.

NEURAL TUNIC (RETINA)

This is the innermost layer of the eye and consists of a thin outer layer that is known as the pigmented part and a thicker inner layer called the neural part. The pigmented part of the retina absorbs light passing through the neural part; this prevents it from reflecting back and causing visual echoes. The neural part of the retina contains light receptors and support cells and is responsible for the preliminary processing and integration of visual information.

ORGANISATION OF THE RETINA

Figure 1.4 illustrates the two types of receptor cells that are found in the outermost layer of the retina, closest to the pigmented part. These receptor cells are known as photoreceptors, which detect light.

- Rods: These photoreceptors do not distinguish between colours. They are highly sensitive and enable vision in very low light levels. Rods are primarily concentrated in a band around the periphery of the retina, with their density decreasing towards the centre of the eye.

- Cones: These photoreceptors provide colour vision and they produce sharper, clearer images than rods, but they require more intense light. Cones are mainly located in the macula lutea, particularly at its centre in an area that is called the fovea.

The elongated outer segments of the rods and cones contain hundreds to thousands of flattened membranous discs. In rods, these discs are separate and form a cylindrical shape. In cones, the discs are folds of the plasma membrane and the outer segment tapers to a blunt point.

COLOUR VISION AND RETINAL STRUCTURE

There are three types of cones – red, blue and green. Colour discrimination relies on the integration of information from these three types of cones. The perception of yellow, for example, occurs when green cones are highly stimulated, red cones are less strongly stimulated and the blue cones have minimal stimulation.

A narrow connecting stalk links the outer segment of a photoreceptor to its inner segment, which contains all of the typical cellular organelles. The inner segment is also where synapses with other cells occur and the neurotransmitters are released.

Rods and cones synapse with neurones called bipolar cells, which in turn synapse with a layer of neurones called ganglion cells. At these synapse points, associated cells can stimulate or inhibit communication between the two cells, altering the retina's sensitivity to different light levels.

- Rods and cones: These are cells located in the retina that detect light.

- Bipolar cells: They receive signals from rods and cones at connection points called synapses.

- Ganglion cells: Bipolar cells pass the signals to these neurones through more synapses.

- Associated cells: Between these connections, other cells can either boost or reduce the signals.

- Adjusting sensitivity: These associated cells help the retina adapt to different levels of light by changing how strong the signals are.

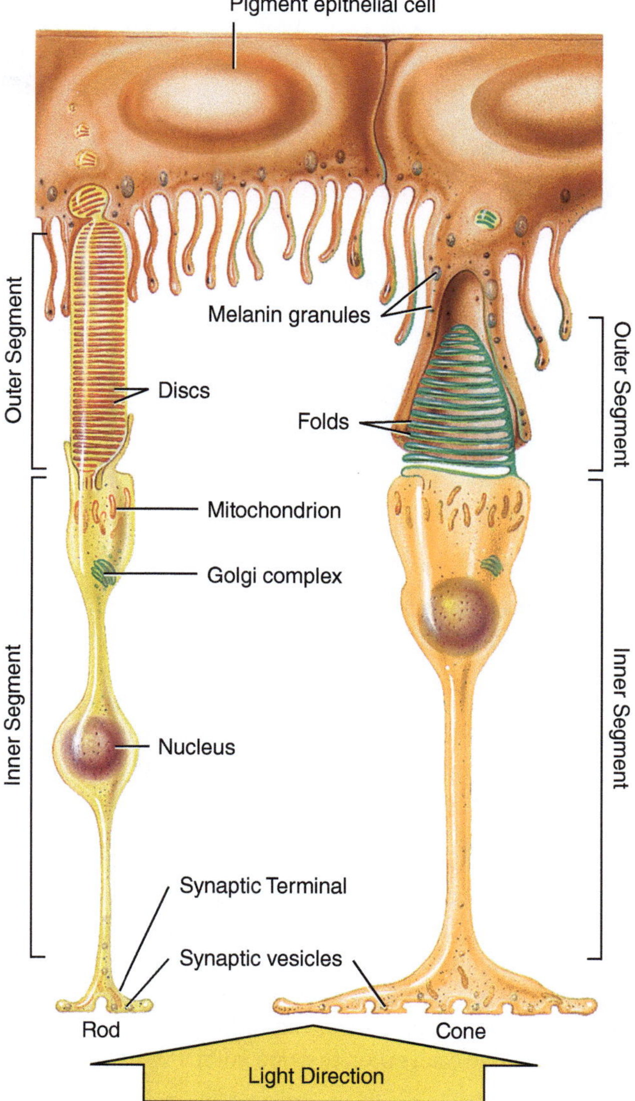

FIGURE 1.4   Cross-section of the retina

In essence, rods and cones pass information to bipolar cells, which then relay it to ganglion cells. Other cells at these connections influence how well the retina responds to light variations (see Figure 1.5).

Axons from approximately one million ganglion cells converge at the optic disc, where they turn, penetrate the wall of the eye and continue to the diencephalon of the brain as the optic nerve. The central retinal artery and vein pass through the centre of the optic nerve. The optic disc lacks photoreceptors, making it a blind spot. We do not notice this blind spot, however, because involuntary eye movements keep the visual image moving, allowing the brain to fill in the missing information.

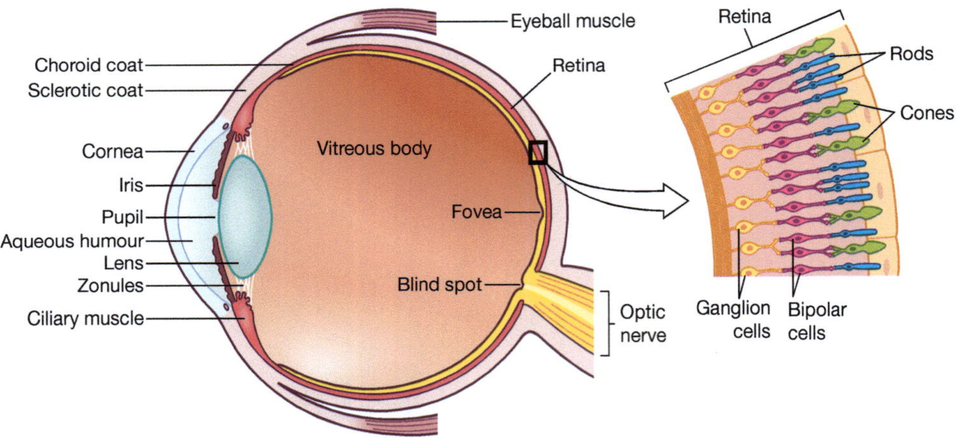

FIGURE 1.5 Rods and cones

EYE CHAMBERS

The eye is divided into two main cavities: a large posterior cavity and a smaller anterior cavity. The anterior cavity further divides into the anterior chamber and the posterior chamber (see Figure 1.3).

The anterior chamber contains a fluid called aqueous humour, which circulates between the anterior and posterior chambers by passing through the pupil. Aqueous humour plays a crucial role as a transport medium for nutrients and waste products. The fluid pressure created by aqueous humour helps maintain the eye's shape. It is produced by epithelial cells in the ciliary body and drains through the canal of Schlemm to the sclera for recycling.

The posterior cavity, which is the larger of the two, is filled with a gel-like substance that is known as vitreous humour. Vitreous humour stabilises the eye's shape against the forces exerted by extraocular muscles. Unlike aqueous humour, vitreous humour forms during eye development and remains unchanged throughout life. A thin layer of aqueous humour bathes the posterior chamber, supplying nutrients to the retina and aiding in waste removal. The pressure it exerts also keeps the neural part of the retina against the pigmented part; while these layers are closely situated to each other, they are not firmly attached to each other, necessitating this external pressure.

FOCUSING IMAGES ON THE RETINA

For a visual image to be clear and usable, it must be focused precisely onto the retina; this is a task that is accomplished by the eye's lens. Initially, the light that enters the eye undergoes refraction and the lens then further adjusts this refraction to ensure that the image is focused precisely on the retina.

REFRACTION

Refraction occurs when the light transitions from one medium to another of differing density (see Figure 1.6).

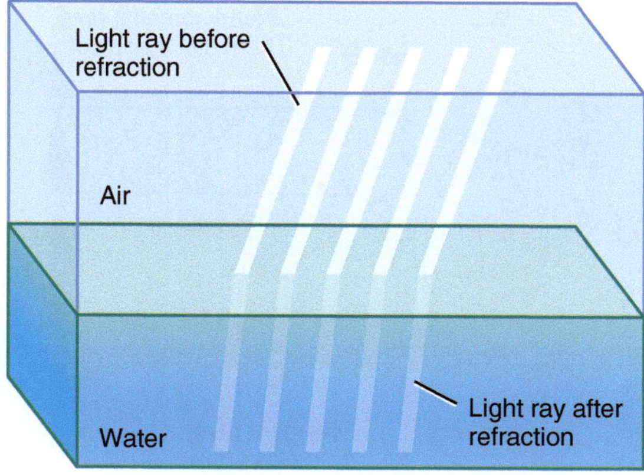

FIGURE 1.6   Refraction of light passing from air (less dense) to water (dense)

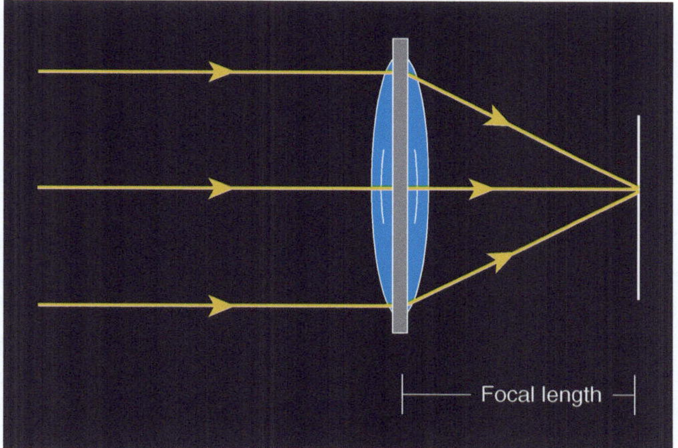

FIGURE 1.7   Focal length

The majority of light refraction in the eye occurs as the light enters the cornea from the air. Additional refraction happens when light passes from the aqueous humour into the lens. The lens provides further refraction to focus light precisely onto the retina, and it can adjust this refraction to accommodate different focal lengths.

FOCAL LENGTH

Focal length refers to the distance between the focal point (such as on the retina) and the centre of the lens (see Figure 1.7). It depends on:

- The distance from the object to the lens: Objects farther away result in shorter focal lengths.

- The shape of the lens: A more curved (rounder) lens causes greater refraction. A very curved lens has a shorter focal length compared to a flatter lens.

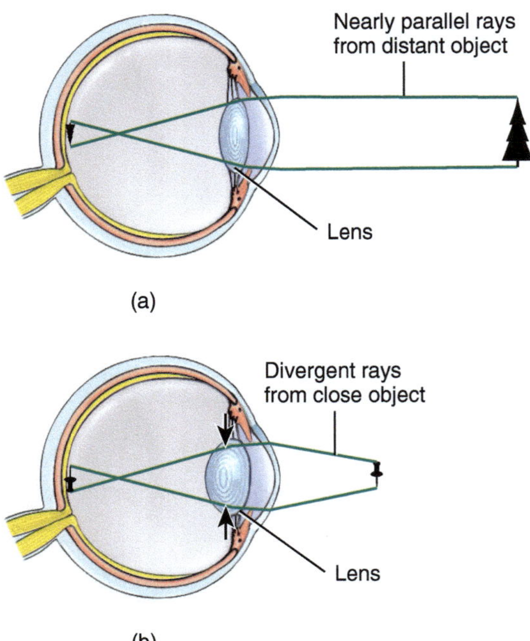

FIGURE 1.8   Accommodation to (a) viewing distant (far) object and (b) viewing close (near) object

The lens is positioned behind the cornea; it is held in place by ligaments that are attached to the ciliary body. It consists of concentric layers of precisely organised cells that are covered by a fibrous capsule. Many of these capsule fibres are elastic, which would naturally make the lens spherical if not for the external forces exerted by the ligaments. Inside the lens are lens fibres, which are specialised cells lacking a nucleus and other organelles. They are filled with a protein called crystallin, essential for the transparency and focusing ability of the lens.

The process of altering the shape of the lens to focus an image onto the retina is known as accommodation. This shape change is controlled by the smooth muscles within the ciliary body, which adjust tension on the suspensory ligaments (see Figure 1.8).

MYOPIA, HYPEROPIA AND PRESBYOPIA

In individuals with myopia (short-sightedness), the lens fails to focus the image directly onto the retina, this causes the focal point to fall in front of it (see Figure 1.9). As a result, those people with myopia can see nearby objects clearly, but distant objects appear blurred. Myopia can be effectively corrected using corrective lenses, such as glasses or contact lenses.

In individuals with hyperopia (long-sightedness), the image is focused onto a point behind the retina (Figure 1.10); therefore, these people can see things at a distance but not those close to them.

Presbyopia is the gradual inability to focus on close objects as people age, primarily due to the reduced elasticity of the lens (see Chapter 8 of this book). This loss affects everyone but varies in onset and impact on vision. Most people notice the onset of presbyopia between 40 and 50 years of age. Corrective glasses, often referred to as reading glasses but beneficial for all near-vision tasks, effectively treat presbyopia.

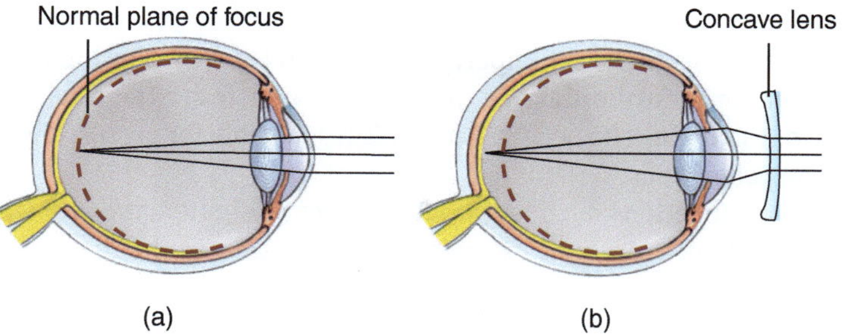

FIGURE 1.9   Near-sighted (myopic) eye (a) uncorrected and (b) corrected by a concave lens

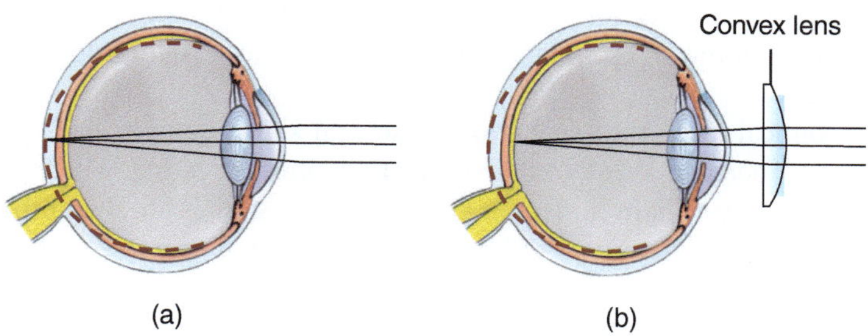

FIGURE 1.10   Long-sighted (hyperopic) eye (a) uncorrected and (b) corrected by a convex lens

PROCESSING OF VISUAL INFORMATION

Ganglion cells, monitoring rods in the retina (M cells), transmit information about the general form of objects, motion and shadows in low-light conditions. Up to 1000 rods may feed into a single M cell, resulting in a loss of specific information; activation of an M cell indicates light has hit a broad area rather than a precise point. However, M cells compensate for this by varying activity based on the pattern of stimulation within their receptive field (area of retina). For example, stimulation at the edge versus the centre of their field elicits different responses.

In contrast, cone cells exhibit minimal convergence. In the fovea, the ratio of cones to ganglion cells is 1 : 1. Ganglion cells monitoring cones (P cells) are more abundant than M cells and, because of minimal convergence, they provide precise, location-specific information. Therefore, cones convey more detailed information about visual images compared to rods.

CENTRAL PROCESSING OF VISUAL INFORMATION

After light stimulates the photoreceptor cells in the retina (rods and cones), the resulting signals are transmitted via specialised neurones called ganglion cells. These ganglion cell axons converge at the back of the eye and exit through the optic disc, collectively forming the optic nerves, known as cranial nerve II.

Upon exiting the eye, these optic nerves travel towards the brain, where their pathways intersect at a crucial junction that is known as the optic chiasm. At the optic chiasm, fibres from each optic nerve split into two groups: one group stays on the same side of the brain, while the other group crosses over to the opposite side.

The fibres that remain on the same side continue to the lateral geniculate nucleus (LGN), located in the thalamus – an important sensory relay centre in the brain. From the LGN, visual information is further relayed to the occipital cortex of the cerebral hemisphere on the same side of the brain. The occipital cortex is responsible for processing visual stimuli and forming visual perceptions.

Simultaneously, functions such as pupillary reflexes – automatic adjustments of the pupil in response to changes in light intensity – are managed in the diencephalon (which includes the thalamus) and brainstem. These regions coordinate involuntary eye movements and responses to visual stimuli.

CONCLUSION

The human eye is composed of impressive anatomical and physiological complexity, reflecting an intricate design that allows for the perception of light and the formation of images. Understanding the anatomy and physiology of the eye provides insight into how we perceive the world around us.

At the anatomical level, the eye comprises several key structures, each playing a vital role in vision. The cornea and lens focus incoming light onto the retina, where photoreceptor cells, rods and cones convert light into neural signals. These signals are then processed by the retina's complex network of neurones and transmitted via the optic nerve to the brain, where visual perception occurs.

Physiologically, vision involves a series of coordinated events starting from the refraction of light as it enters the eye, the accommodation of the lens to adjust focus and the phototransduction process in the retina. The rods and cones play a critical role in detecting light intensity and colour, respectively, enabling both low-light and daylight vision. The brain's visual cortex integrates these signals to create a coherent visual representation of our surroundings.

The eye's ability to adapt to varying light conditions, maintain focus on objects at different distances and perceive a wide range of colours highlights its remarkable functional capabilities. Disorders of the eye, such as myopia, hyperopia, cataracts and glaucoma, highlight the importance of each component in maintaining optimal vision.

When sight becomes impaired, it profoundly impacts an individual's quality of life. Vision impairment can result from a variety of causes, including genetic factors, age-related changes, injuries or diseases. Conditions such as macular degeneration, diabetic retinopathy and retinal detachment disrupt the normal functioning of the eye's components, leading to partial or complete loss of vision. Early detection and advances in treatments and technologies are key in managing these conditions and preventing further vision loss.

The eye's anatomy and physiology are central to our understanding of sight. This knowledge not only enhances our appreciation of this critical sensory organ but also informs medical and technological advances aimed at preserving and restoring vision. Understanding the interplay between the structural and functional aspects of the eye continues to be an important area of study in both health and disease.

GLOSSARY OF TERMS

Accommodation: The process by which the eye's lens changes shape to focus on objects at various distances.

Aqueous humour: The clear fluid filling the space in the front of the eyeball between the lens and the cornea.

Choroid: The vascular layer of the eye containing connective tissues and lying between the retina and the sclera.

Ciliary body: A ring of tissue behind the iris that is involved in changing the shape of the lens (accommodation) and producing aqueous humour.

Cone cells: Photoreceptor cells in the retina responsible for colour vision and high spatial acuity.

Cornea: The transparent front part of the eye that covers the iris, pupil and anterior chamber and is involved in light refraction.

Fovea: A small depression in the retina where visual acuity is highest, located in the centre of the macula.

Hyperopia: Also known as farsightedness, a condition where distant objects are seen more clearly than near objects.

Iris: The coloured part of the eye, which controls the size of the pupil and thus the amount of light that enters the eye.

Lens: A transparent, biconvex structure in the eye that helps to refract light to be focused on the retina.

Macula: The central area of the retina responsible for detailed central vision.

Myopia: Also known as near-sightedness, a condition where near objects are seen more clearly than distant objects.

Optic nerve: The nerve that transmits visual information from the retina to the brain.

Photoreceptors: Specialised cells in the retina (rods and cones) that convert light into electrical signals.

Pupil: The opening in the centre of the iris that allows light to enter the eye.

Retina: The light-sensitive layer at the back of the eye that contains photoreceptors and converts light into neural signals.

Rod cells: Photoreceptor cells in the retina responsible for vision in low-light conditions.

Sclera: The white, outer layer of the eyeball, providing structure and protection.

Vitreous humour: The clear gel that fills the space between the lens and the retina in the eyeball.

MULTIPLE CHOICE QUESTIONS

1. Which part of the eye is responsible for focusing light onto the retina?
   a) Iris
   b) Lens
   c) Cornea
   d) Sclera

2. What is the function of rod cells in the retina?
   a) Detecting colour
   b) Detecting light intensity and motion
   c) Focusing light
   d) Producing aqueous humour

3. Which part of the eye adjusts the size of the pupil?
   a) Lens
   b) Cornea
   c) Retina
   d) Iris

4. What is the clear, gel-like substance that fills the space between the lens and the retina?
   a) Aqueous humour
   b) Vitreous humour
   c) Sclera
   d) Choroid

5. Where is the highest concentration of cone cells found in the retina?
   a) Optic disc
   b) Peripheral retina
   c) Fovea
   d) Macula

6. Which structure connects the retina to the brain?
   a) Ciliary body
   b) Optic nerve
   c) Macula
   d) Choroid

7. What is the main function of the cornea?
   a) Adjusting the size of the pupil
   b) Refracting light to help focus it on the retina
   c) Producing tears
   d) Nourishing the eye with blood supply

8. Which condition is also known as farsightedness?
   a) Myopia
   b) Hyperopia
   c) Astigmatism
   d) Presbyopia

9. Which cells in the retina are responsible for colour vision?
   a) Rod cells
   b) Cone cells
   c) Ganglion cells
   d) Bipolar cells

10. Which structure produces the aqueous humour?
    a) Retina
    b) Ciliary body
    c) Lens
    d) Choroid

REFERENCES

Clare, C. (2020). The senses (Chapter 15). In: *Fundamentals of Anatomy and Physiology*, 3e (eds. I. Peate and S. Evans). Oxford: Wiley.

Sanderson, A. (2019). Nursing patients with disorders of the eye and sight impairment (Chapter 14). In: *Alexander's Nursing Practice*, 5e (ed. I. Peate). London: Elsevier.

 # Assessment of the Eyes

Humans are highly visual creatures, relying extensively on their sense of sight to navigate, understand and interact with the world around them. Our brains are wired to process visual information rapidly and efficiently, allowing us to recognise faces, interpret emotions and read body language. Visual stimuli often have a profound impact on our emotions, memories and decision-making processes. This reliance on vision shapes many aspects of our lives, from how we communicate and learn. Assessing a patient's vision is a critical component of healthcare that goes beyond merely evaluating their ability to see. A comprehensive vision assessment enables healthcare providers to devise personalised care plans that address both immediate and long-term needs, ensuring optimal patient outcomes.

IMPORTANCE OF VISION ASSESSMENT

IDENTIFYING POTENTIAL RISKS

A thorough vision assessment helps in identifying any risks that are associated with impaired sight. Patients with reduced visual acuity are more prone to accidents such as falls, which can lead to serious injuries, particularly in the elderly. By recognising these risks early, we can assist in the implementation of preventive measures, such as environmental modifications, to reduce the likelihood of accidents.

ENSURING A SAFE ENVIRONMENT

Maintaining a safe environment for patients with impaired vision is paramount. Simple changes, such as ensuring adequate lighting, removing trip hazards and using contrasting colours for better visual differentiation, can significantly enhance safety. For those patients who are in hospital or those in care facilities, these adjustments are essential to prevent incidents that could compromise their health and well-being.

PRESERVING INDEPENDENCE

Vision plays a crucial role in a person's ability to perform daily activities independently. Tasks such as reading, driving, cooking and personal grooming all rely heavily on visual input. Assessing and addressing vision problems can help maintain a patient's independence, enhancing their quality of life. For instance, providing magnifying aids, large print materials or assistive technologies can enable individuals to continue engaging in their usual activities.

REPORTING CHANGES IN VISUAL ACUITY

Any significant changes in a patient's visual acuity must be promptly reported to an appropriate health and care provider. Such changes could indicate the progression of underlying conditions including glaucoma (see Chapter 3 of this book), macular degeneration or diabetic retinopathy, which require immediate attention to prevent further deterioration. Timely intervention can halt or slow the progression of these conditions, preserving as much vision as possible.

COMPREHENSIVE CARE PLANNING

Integrating vision assessment into the overall care plan can address both the physical and psychological impacts of vision loss. This holistic approach ensures that patients receive the support they need to adapt to their visual impairments. It includes:

- Referring patients to vision rehabilitation specialists who can teach adaptive techniques and the use of assistive devices.

- Providing access to counselling services and support groups to help patients cope with the emotional impact of vision loss.

- Scheduling regular follow-ups to monitor vision changes and adjust care plans as necessary.

COLLABORATIVE APPROACH

A multidisciplinary approach is often required to manage vision impairment effectively. Collaboration among ophthalmologists, optometrists, occupational therapists and primary care providers ensures a comprehensive evaluation and management strategy. This team approach ensures that all aspects of the patient's vision health are addressed, from diagnosis and treatment to rehabilitation and support.

THE ASSESSMENT

Assessing a patient's vision is essential for planning appropriate care, ensuring safety and maintaining independence. Recognising and addressing vision changes promptly can prevent further complications and enhance the patient's quality of life. A proactive and holistic approach, involving a multidisciplinary team, ensures that patients receive the best possible care tailored to their unique needs.

Given the critical role of vision in human functioning, assessing a patient's vision is an important component of healthcare (Needham 2019). A comprehensive vision assessment goes beyond simply determining visual acuity (i.e. the ability to see clearly). It encompasses several dimensions:

- Visual acuity: This measures the sharpness of vision and is typically assessed using eye charts. It helps in identifying refractive errors (these occur when the eye cannot properly focus light on the retina, leading to blurred vision) such as myopia (near-sightedness), hyperopia (farsightedness) and astigmatism (a condition where vision is blurred at any distance).

- Visual field testing: This evaluates the range of vision, detecting issues such as peripheral vision loss, which can indicate glaucoma or other neurological conditions.

- Colour vision testing: This assesses the ability to distinguish colours, identifying conditions such as colour blindness (see Box 2.1).

- Depth perception: This evaluates the ability to perceive the world in three dimensions and judge distances accurately. This ability is important for performing everyday tasks and navigating the environment safely. It involves the brain integrating information from both eyes (binocular vision) and other visual cues to create a sense of depth and spatial relationships.

- Eye health examination: This includes a thorough examination of the eye's anatomy, including the cornea, lens, retina and optic nerve, to detect diseases such as cataracts, macular degeneration and diabetic retinopathy.

- Binocular vision: This assesses the ability of the eyes to work together, detecting issues such as strabismus (misalignment of the eyes) and amblyopia (lazy eye). Effective binocular vision allows for accurate depth perception and a wider field of view, which are essential for various daily activities and overall visual perception. The assessment of binocular vision is essential to detect and diagnose any abnormalities that might affect the coordination and function of the eyes.

BOX 2.1   COLOUR BLINDNESS

Colour vision relies on the normal functioning of the retinal cones. Colour blindness does not equate to complete blindness. In fact, many people with colour blindness are unaware of their condition until they undergo a colour vision test. A person with colour blindness cannot distinguish between certain colours, typically red and green. Approximately 8% of the male population is born with colour vision deficiencies, compared to only about 1% of females. Colour blindness can be congenital or acquired due to conditions such as optic neuritis or drug dependency.

The most common method for testing colour vision is the use of Ishihara colour-dotted plates. With advancing technology, there are also apps and electronic tools available for screening colour blindness. Individuals with colour vision defects cannot distinguish the numbers from the surrounding background on these plates. Certain professions, such as pilots and electricians, require normal colour vision for safety reasons. However, there are no driving restrictions for colour-blind individuals since traffic lights have a fixed sequence that can be recognised by position rather than colour.

Source: Adapted from Sanderson (2019); Galloway et al. (2022).

Gibbons (2019) reports that the purpose of examining the eye is to assess the function of the eye and its anatomy and to discern pathology that affects vision. Sanderson (2019) notes it is essential to understand the appearance of a normal eye and the typical recovery process that occurs after surgery or disease. A systematic examination of the eye, using a good light source and methodically inspecting all ocular structures from the outermost to the innermost, is essential. Adopting this approach helps in identifying abnormalities. Table 2.1 itemises the clinical features that may be observed during an eye examination and their possible implications.

Previously, patients with eye conditions were typically referred to specialist eye centres. However, an increasing number of clinicians are now evaluating ophthalmic conditions in various settings, such as outreach centres, emergency departments, walk-in centres and general practice settings. Assessing the eye is important. According to the Royal National Institute of Blind People, there are over two million people in the UK living with sight loss. There are 320 000 people registered as blind or partially sighted; nearly 80% are 65 years or older, and approximately 60% are 75 years plus. Age is a significant risk factor related to eye health and sight loss (Royal National Institute of Blind People 2021).

Table 2.1   Clinical findings from an eye examination

Structure	Clinical features	Significance
Lids	Bruising (ecchymosis) Swelling Drooping (ptosis) Increased lacrimation Discharge	• Surgical handling • Trauma • Infection
Conjunctiva	Redness (injection; see Figure 2.1) Swelling (chemosis)	• Surgical handling • Trauma • Allergy • Infection
Cornea	Cloudy Crinkled Fluorescein staining Suture line not intact Penetrating injury	• Increased intraocular pressure • Infection • Loss of anterior chamber • Ulceration
Anterior chamber	Hyphaema (blood in anterior chamber) Hypopyon (pus in anterior chamber) Shallow anterior chamber	• Hyphaema due to surgery should gradually resolve • Increasing intraocular pressure indicates bleeding/inflammation • Hypopyon indicates infection • Shallow may indicate aqueous loss
Iris Pupil	Muddy Irregular shape	• Inflammation • Iris prolapse • Adhesions • Trauma

Source: Adapted from Sanderson (2019); Gibbons (2019).

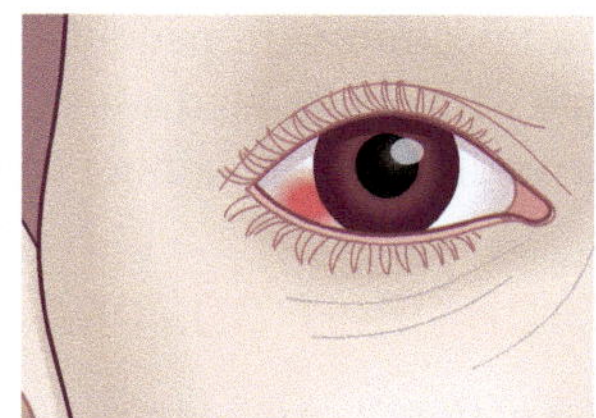

FIGURE 2.1   Redness

PATIENT HISTORY IN OPHTHALMIC ASSESSMENT

Gathering a patient history provides valuable insight into how the patient perceives their own vision and overall eye health. It permits an understanding of the patient's personal experience with their vision, including any changes or symptoms they have noticed. By discussing their daily visual challenges, including any difficulties with tasks such as reading or seeing at a distance and their overall visual comfort, it enables those who offer care and support to better assess the impact of vision problems on the patient's quality of life. This comprehensive understanding helps in diagnosing potential issues, tailoring treatment plans and providing more effective care based on the patient's specific needs and concerns.

When examining a patient with an ophthalmic condition, it is crucial to follow a logical and systematic approach to history taking, visual assessment, examination and diagnosis. Failing to use this structured approach may result in missing critical signs and symptoms.

Patients with symptoms related to their eyes may feel anxious and need sensitivity and understanding during their examination. It is crucial for the examiner to maintain a calm and confident demeanour. If patients are not treated with friendliness and professionalism, they may hold back some of their concerns (Jarvis and Eckhradt 2024; Rhoads and Wiggins Petersen 2021).

DOCUMENTATION OF FINDINGS

When conducting a history-gathering exercise for individuals with eye-related issues, clear documentation is paramount. This ensures that all relevant symptoms, patient history and observations are accurately recorded, facilitating an accurate diagnosis. Comprehensive records allow those who offer care and support to people to consider all details and nuances of the patient's condition, leading to a more precise understanding and development of a treatment plan.

Clear documentation is also crucial for maintaining consistent care, particularly when multiple healthcare providers are involved. It ensures that each provider can quickly grasp the patient's history, previous treatments and current condition, thereby promoting a seamless and coordinated approach to patient care.

Tracking the progress of the patient over time is another significant benefit of clear documentation. By recording changes in the patient's condition, this can help to evaluate the effectiveness of treatments, make necessary adjustments and promptly address any worsening symptoms. This ongoing record is essential for optimising patient outcomes.

High-quality notes and documentation serve as legal records of the patient's condition and the care provided. This is important for both patient and provider protection in case of disputes or legal issues. It also facilitates better communication with the patient, helping them understand their condition and treatment plans. This understanding can improve concordance (adherence) to treatment and overall satisfaction with the care received.

Clear and thorough documentation is essential for accurate diagnosis, consistent and coordinated care, effective communication with patients, legal accountability and error prevention in the treatment of people with eye-related issues.

The following features are required when gaining a patient history.

PRESENTING COMPLAINT (OR CHIEF COMPLAINT OF PRESENT ILLNESS)

The first step is to understand the patient's chief complaint and to determine why the patient has attended. Patients might present with various symptoms such as vision loss, eye pain, redness, floaters, flashes of light, photophobia or double vision. Understanding the primary issue sets the direction for further questions. It is important to ask detailed questions about these symptoms:

- Onset: When did the symptoms begin? Was the onset sudden or gradual? Sudden onset might suggest acute conditions such as retinal detachment or vascular occlusions, whereas gradual onset may point to chronic conditions, for example, cataracts or glaucoma.

- Duration: How long have the symptoms been present? Duration can help differentiate between acute and chronic conditions.

- Severity: How severe are the symptoms? Are they worsening, improving or fluctuating? Determining severity can impact urgency and treatment choices.

- Associated factors: Are there any triggers or activities that worsen or alleviate the symptoms, for example, headache, nausea or systemic symptoms?

- Previous episodes: Has the patient experienced similar symptoms in the past? If there are recurrent symptoms, this may indicate a chronic or recurring condition.

PAST MEDICAL HISTORY

A comprehensive past medical history is essential. Ocular history focuses on:

- Previous eye conditions: Any history of eye diseases such as glaucoma, macular degeneration, uveitis or dry eye syndrome.

- Surgery and injuries: History of ocular surgery (e.g. cataract surgery, laser-assisted in situ keratomileusis [LASIK] can be an alternative to glasses or contact lenses) or trauma.

- Treatments: Previous treatment and their outcomes.

Systemic medical health can significantly impact eye health:

- Chronic conditions: Diabetes, hypertension, thyroid disorders, autoimmune diseases and infectious diseases (e.g. HIV, syphilis) can have ocular manifestations.

- Medications: A detailed list of current and past medications, including over-the-counter drugs and supplements. Some medications have ocular side effects (e.g. corticosteroids, antimalarials).

FAMILY HISTORY

Family history can provide clues about genetic conditions (hereditary) or predispositions to certain eye diseases:

- Ocular diseases: Family history of glaucoma, macular degeneration, retinitis pigmentosa and so on.

- Systemic diseases: Family history of systemic diseases that can affect the eyes.

SOCIAL AND OCCUPATIONAL HISTORY

Understanding the patient's lifestyle and occupation helps in identifying environmental or occupational factors that might affect eye health:

- Occupation: Jobs involving prolonged screen time, exposure to bright lights or potential eye hazards/digital eye strain.

- Lifestyle: Smoking, alcohol consumption and hobbies that may strain the eyes (e.g. extensive reading, screen use).
- Environmental exposure: Exposure to dust, toxic substances, chemicals or allergens.

REVIEW OF SYSTEMS

A systemic review helps to identify related symptoms that might provide additional clues:

- Neurological symptoms: Presence of headaches, dizziness or neurological deficits may indicate a neurological cause of eye symptoms.
- General health: Symptoms such as fatigue, weight loss or fever can indicate systemic diseases affecting the eyes.
- Other sensory symptoms: Changes in hearing or taste might indicate broader systemic involvement.

VISUAL AND FUNCTIONAL HISTORY

Baseline vision: Understanding the patient's baseline visual acuity and any existing visual impairments.

- Corrective lenses: Use of glasses or contact lenses and their prescriptions.
- Previous eye examinations: Results of previous eye examinations and any noted changes over time.

Impact on daily activities: How the symptoms affect daily life, including:

- Reading: Difficulty with reading or seeing fine details.
- Driving: Impact on the ability to drive, particularly at night.
- Occupational tasks: Challenges in performing job-related tasks.

PSYCHOSOCIAL IMPACT

Emotional and mental health: Eye problems can significantly impact a patient's quality of life and mental well-being:

- Emotional impact: Anxiety, depression or stress related to vision problems.
- Support systems: Availability of family or community support.

SUMMARISING AND CLARIFYING

After gathering the history, it is essential to summarise the key points to ensure nothing important has been missed. This involves repeating back to the patient the main aspects of their history to confirm accuracy and completeness. Clarifying any ambiguous information helps in forming a clear clinical picture.

Taking a detailed history in patients with eye problems is an integral part of the diagnostic process. This involves understanding the chief complaint, past medical and family history, social and occupational factors, a review of systems, visual and functional history and the psychosocial impact of the eye problems. This comprehensive approach ensures that all relevant information is gathered, aiding in accurate diagnosis and effective treatment planning. Clear and thorough documentation is essential for providing high-quality, consistent care.

After taking a comprehensive history from a patient with eye problems, the next steps involve a systematic clinical examination, appropriate diagnostic tests and formulation of a management plan.

TESTING VISUAL FUNCTION

Prior to undertaking any physical examination, it is imperative to adhere to local policies and procedures regarding consent, the provision of a chaperone and the implementation of infection control and prevention strategies.

When examining the eye, it is important to start from the outside and work inwards. Begin by observing the patient's face as a whole to check for facial symmetry and any obvious signs such as palsy, ptosis (drooping of the eyelid; see Figure 2.2), proptosis (bulging of the eye) or allergic reactions. Take into account the patient's age and psychological condition, as these factors can influence the examination process. For example, patients with Parkinson's disease might have difficulty positioning themselves for a slit-lamp examination (Gibbons 2019).

Start the examination by asking the patient to open both eyes, as this is typically easier than opening one eye at a time. If a slit lamp is not available, a good pen torch or magnifying light is essential for inspecting the eye and assessing pupil reactions (see Box 2.2). If the patient is in pain, local anaesthetic drops may be necessary before proceeding with the examination. However, if there is a glass foreign body present, or if the patient has a history suggesting a possible penetrating injury or perforation from drilling or high-speed equipment, avoid using local anaesthetic (Gibbons 2019). These cases require immediate referral to an eye unit or ophthalmic emergency department, both day and night. Do not apply any pressure or padding to the eye; instead, use a Cartella eye shield, a transparent plastic shield designed to protect the eye and prevent further injury after operations.

If the patient reports a foreign body sensation but no foreign body is visible on the cornea, it is crucial to evert the upper eyelid to inspect underneath. Use fluorescein eye drops to highlight any scratches or abrasions on the eye (Gibbons 2019).

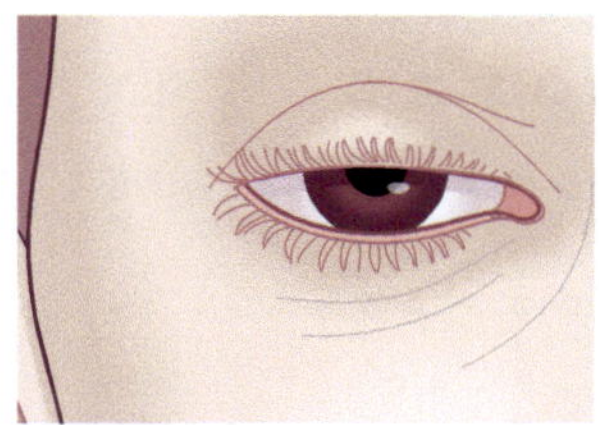

FIGURE 2.2   Ptosis

BOX 2.2	ASSESSING PUPIL SIZE AND REACTIVITY

The size, shape and reactivity of pupils should be assessed as part of an eye examination. The procedure should be explained to the patient and the patient asked to keep their eyes open. Wash hands. Gently hold the eyelid open if this is required. Using a pen torch, shine the light across the pupil, observing for it to constrict briskly as the light passes. The opposite eye should show constriction at the same time. Wash hands. It may be difficult to detect pupil constriction in patients with dark irises. Ensuring the overhead lights are dimmed may aid this. Report and document findings.

Source: Adapted from O'Driscoll (2022).

VISUAL ACUITY

Obtaining an accurate visual acuity assessment is important, as it establishes a baseline of the patient's vision and forms the foundation for clinical decision-making regarding treatment options. Visual acuity is the quantitative or mathematical measurement of visual function at various distances. It enables a measurement of what the patient can see in a more objective manner.

Distance Vision Distance vision is tested using Snellen test-type charts, which display letters or pictures that are arranged in rows of precise and diminishing size (see Figure 2.3). Each eye should be tested separately, with the benefit, if worn, of any spectacles or contact

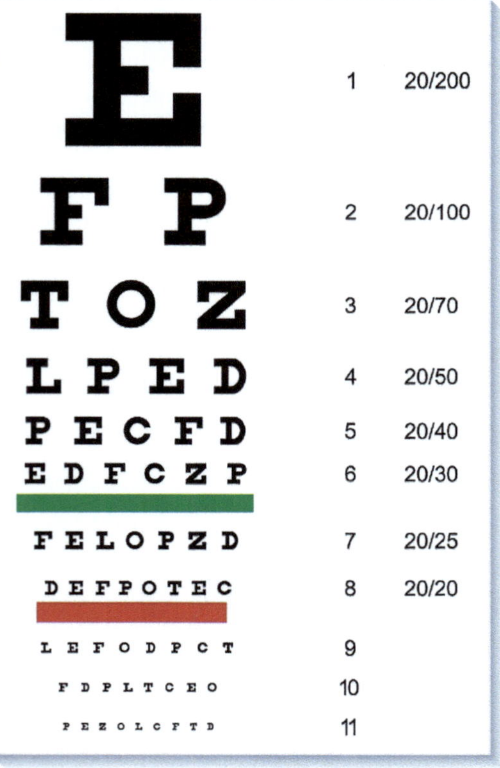

FIGURE 2.3 Snellen chart

lenses, to ensure that 'best corrected vision' is being checked (Phillips 2023). The eye not being tested must be completely occluded. In normal testing, patients are positioned 6 m away from the chart and asked to read each line aloud, until they can no longer make out the letters. The result is recorded as a fraction of the distance from the chart in metres over the normal reading distance of the last complete line read, plus the number of extra letters read from the line below or minus the number of letters read incorrectly, e.g. 6/9 − 2 (Figure 2.3). If glasses or contact lenses are worn, this is also recorded.

LogMAR VISION TESTING

Although more complex, LogMAR vision testing is recognised for its accuracy in measuring visual acuity (Galloway et al. 2022). The primary advantage of a LogMAR chart is that each line contains five letters and each letter is scored, providing a more equitable assessment of the patient's ability to read the letters. The main drawback for the tester is that it can be time-consuming initially and clinicians may be discouraged by the need to calculate individual scores. However, most departments use a conversion chart to simplify recording the patient's score (Royal College of Ophthalmologists 2015). The LogMAR vision chart is mainly used in clinics specialising in low vision, glaucoma and macular degeneration.

TUMBLING 'E', 'E' TEST

Young children, those unable to read and those who do not know the Roman alphabet can be asked to do the tumbling 'E' or 'E' test. Instead of letters or numbers, the chart features the capital letter 'E' in different orientations (rotated by 90°). The patient must indicate the direction in which the arms of the 'E' are pointing (up, down, left or right).

If the patient has learning difficulties, developmental delays, poor concentration or expressive dysphasia, visual acuity testing can be done using a Sheridan–Gardiner singles booklet, where single letters or pictures of varying sizes are presented one at a time, and the patient is asked to match them on a card with a limited choice of symbols (Meakin and Seewoodhary 2022). The test is conducted in a similar way to the Snellen test, but the scoring system for every letter missed is more exact.

Normal distance visual acuity is considered to be 6/6. If a patient's vision is less than 6/9 or 6/12 (with variations related to local policy), they should be asked to read the chart again while looking through a pinhole. This method can help determine if the issue is purely a refractive error, as vision should improve with the pinhole by reducing peripheral light stimulation. However, a posterior segment problem, such as age-related macular degeneration, will not improve with pinhole testing. If the patient cannot read the top letter (6/60), further tests include assessing their ability to count fingers at 1 m, detect hand movements or perceive light.

Near Vision   Near-vision testing assesses how well a person can see objects that are close to them, typically within arm's length. This type of vision is crucial for activities such as reading, writing and other tasks that require focus on nearby objects. The test is carried out with good illumination and the patient is asked to read text in various sizes of standard print that are prefixed with the letter N (similar to the Snellen chart). N5 is accepted as normal reading acuity (Sanderson 2019). Near-vision testing is essential for identifying problems such as presbyopia, myopia (near-sightedness) and other conditions that affect a person's ability to perform close-up tasks. Regular testing helps in prescribing appropriate corrective lenses and in monitoring the progression of vision problems.

Binocular Vision The ability to use the eyes together is called binocular vision. Binocular vision testing evaluates how well both eyes work together to provide a single, cohesive visual image and accurate depth perception. This testing is crucial for diagnosing and treating issues such as strabismus (squint/eye misalignment), amblyopia (lazy eye) and other binocular vision anomalies.

The test involves the simultaneous perception of images by both eyes and the fusion of these images in the visual cortex to create a single, cohesive image. Binocular vision is crucial for stereopsis, which is depth perception. Additionally, having two functioning eyes expands the field of vision and eliminates deficits caused by natural blind spots.

The visual field (or perimeter) refers to the range of vision an eye can perceive in terms of angle, rather than distance. Typically, this range is about 60º towards the nose (nasally), 90º towards the temples (temporally), 50º upwards (superiorly) and 70º downwards (inferiorly).

Assessing the visual field is crucial for managing various conditions such as glaucoma, intermittent vision loss, transient ischaemic attacks, strokes (cerebrovascular accidents), neurological diseases and retinal detachment. Visual field assessment is conducted using perimetry in an ophthalmic setting, a method that employs a field analyser to accurately measure visual field defects, known as scotomas (Galloway et al. 2022).

In a primary care environment, a simpler method called the confrontation test is used. The confrontation test is a simple, preliminary method used to assess a patient's visual fields. To perform the test, the examiner and patient sit facing each other, about 1 m apart. The patient covers one eye while the examiner does the same with the opposite eye. The examiner then uses their fingers or a small object, moving it from the periphery towards the centre in each of the four quadrants of the patient's visual field – temporal, nasal, superior and inferior.

The patient is asked to indicate when they first see the examiner's fingers or object. The examiner compares these responses with their own visual field to identify any discrepancies. Abnormalities may indicate visual field defects, such as scotomas or losses in specific areas, necessitating more detailed follow-up testing if significant issues are detected (Borooah and Tint 2023).

COLOUR VISION ASSESSMENT

Colour blindness can be either congenital or acquired through conditions such as optic neuritis or drug dependency (Sanderson 2019). Colour vision assessment should be conducted for any patient who presents with painful vision loss, particularly if an optic nerve condition is suspected or for individuals who request testing for occupational reasons.

The most common method for testing colour vision involves using Ishihara plates, which display numbers within coloured dot patterns. These plates consist of a circle of dots with numbers embedded within the pattern, designed to test for red-green colour blindness. The patient covers one eye and attempts to read the number on each plate. If a number cannot be distinguished, it is subtracted from the total score. For example, if there are 17 plates in total and the patient correctly reads 16 numbers, the result would be recorded as 16/17. This means the patient successfully identified 16 out of 17 numbers.

Advances in technology have introduced apps and electronic tools for colour blindness screening. It should be noted that personal computer display settings, ambient light and other factors can affect test results.

DIAGNOSTIC TESTS

Diagnosing eye conditions accurately often requires a range of diagnostic tests. These tests help to assess the structure and function of various parts of the eye, detect abnormalities and guide treatment decisions. An overview of some commonly used diagnostic tests in ophthalmology is provided in Table 2.2.

Table 2.2 Some diagnostic tests in ophthalmology

Diagnostic test	Discussion
Visual acuity test	Purpose: Measures the sharpness or clarity of vision at various distances.
	Procedure: Patients read letters on a Snellen chart or similar device, covering one eye at a time.
	Applications: Essential for diagnosing refractive errors (myopia, hyperopia, astigmatism) and assessing the impact of eye diseases on vision.
Slit-lamp examination	Purpose: Provides a magnified view of the anterior segment of the eye.
	Procedure: A slit lamp (biomicroscope) illuminates and magnifies the eye structures, including the cornea, lens and anterior chamber.
	Applications: Diagnoses cataracts, corneal ulcers, foreign bodies, conjunctivitis, uveitis and other anterior segment diseases.
Tonometry	Purpose: Measures intraocular pressure.
	Procedure: Several methods exist, including applanation tonometry (e.g. Goldmann tonometer) and non-contact (air puff) tonometry.
	Applications: Critical for diagnosing and managing glaucoma.
Ophthalmoscopy (fundoscopy)	Purpose: Examines the retina, optic disc, macula and retinal blood vessels.
	Procedure: Direct or indirect ophthalmoscope illuminates and magnifies the interior structures of the eye.
	Applications: Detects diabetic retinopathy, macular degeneration, retinal detachment, optic neuritis and other posterior segment conditions.
Optical coherence tomography	Purpose: Provides high-resolution cross-sectional images of the retina and optic nerve head.
	Procedure: Non-invasive imaging technique that uses light waves to take detailed pictures of the retina.
	Applications: Diagnoses macular degeneration, diabetic retinopathy, macular holes, retinal oedema and glaucoma.
Fluorescein angiography	Purpose: Visualises blood flow in the retina and choroid.
	Procedure: Intravenous injection of fluorescein dye followed by a series of photographs using a specialised camera.
	Applications: Diagnoses and monitors diabetic retinopathy, macular degeneration, retinal vein occlusion and other retinal vascular diseases.

(Continued)

Table 2.2 (*Continued*)

Diagnostic test	Discussion
Amsler grid	Purpose: Detects abnormalities in the central visual field.
	Procedure: Patients view a grid pattern and report any distortions, missing areas or wavy lines.
	Applications: Screening tool for macular degeneration and other macular disorders.
Ultrasound biomicroscopy	Purpose: Visualises the anterior segment structures in high detail.
	Procedure: High-frequency ultrasound probe scans the anterior segment of the eye.
	Applications: Useful in opaque media, assessing anterior segment tumours, angle-closure glaucoma and iris abnormalities.
Corneal topography	Purpose: Maps the curvature of the cornea.
	Procedure: A computer-assisted device creates a topographic map of the cornea's surface.
	Applications: Diagnoses keratoconus, evaluates corneal astigmatism and assists in planning refractive surgery.
Electrodiagnostic testing	Electroretinography:
	Purpose: Measures the electrical response of the retina's photoreceptors (rods and cones).
	Procedure: Electrodes are placed on the cornea and skin around the eye and light stimuli are used to elicit retinal responses.
	Applications: Diagnoses retinitis pigmentosa, cone-rod dystrophies and other retinal disorders.
	Visual evoked potentials:
	Purpose: Assesses the electrical activity in the visual cortex in response to visual stimuli.
	Procedure: Electrodes are placed on the scalp and visual stimuli (e.g. flashing lights or patterns) are presented.
	Applications: Detects optic neuropathies, demyelinating diseases such as multiple sclerosis and visual pathway disorders.
Fundus photography	Purpose: Captures detailed images of the retina, optic disc and macula.
	Procedure: Specialised cameras take photographs of the back of the eye.
	Applications: Documentation and monitoring of retinal diseases, diabetic retinopathy and macular degeneration.
Pachymetry	Purpose: Measures the thickness of the cornea.
	Procedure: Uses ultrasonic or optical devices to measure corneal thickness.
	Applications: Important in assessing corneal health, diagnosing corneal oedema and preoperative evaluation for refractive surgery.

Diagnostic test	Discussion
Gonioscopy	Purpose: Examines the anterior chamber angle where the iris meets the cornea.
	Procedure: A special lens (goniolens) is placed on the eye and a slit lamp is used to view the angle.
	Applications: Diagnoses different types of glaucoma, including angle-closure glaucoma and secondary glaucomas.
Specular microscopy	Purpose: Analyses the endothelial cell layer of the cornea.
	Procedure: Non-invasive imaging technique that captures detailed images of the corneal endothelium.
	Applications: Assesses endothelial cell density and morphology, important for diagnosing and managing corneal diseases and evaluating suitability for corneal transplantation.

Source: Adapted from Galloway et al. (2022), Sanderson (2019) and Meakin and Seewoodhary (2022).

The diagnostic tests highlighted in Table 2.2 are essential tools in the evaluation and management of various eye conditions. They provide detailed insight into the anatomy and function of the eye, helping those who offer care and support to patients with eye conditions to diagnose them accurately, monitor disease progression and plan effective treatments. Each test has specific applications and is chosen based on the patient's symptoms, history and initial examination findings.

CONCLUSION

Assessing a patient with eye conditions requires a comprehensive and systematic approach that integrates detailed history taking, thorough clinical examination and appropriate diagnostic testing. The process begins with understanding the patient's symptoms, medical history and lifestyle factors, followed by a meticulous examination of the eye's various structures using tools such as visual acuity tests, slit-lamp biomicroscopy and ophthalmoscopy.

Diagnostic tests such as optical coherence tomography, visual field testing and fluorescein angiography provide critical insights into specific eye conditions, enabling precise diagnosis and effective treatment planning. Other specialised tests such as tonometry for intraocular pressure measurement, corneal topography and electrodiagnostic testing further enhance the ability to diagnose and manage complex eye diseases.

The integration of these steps ensures a holistic assessment, allowing for accurate diagnosis, tailored treatment plans and continuous monitoring of the patient's condition. Clear documentation and effective communication with the patient and other healthcare providers are essential to ensure continuity of care and optimal outcomes.

Ultimately, a thorough and methodical approach to assessing patients with eye conditions is crucial for preserving and improving vision, enhancing quality of life and preventing potential complications.

GLOSSARY OF TERMS

Amsler grid: A tool used to detect visual disturbances caused by macular degeneration or other central retinal issues.

Biomicroscopy (slit-lamp examination): A technique using a slit lamp to examine the anterior segment of the eye in detail.

Blind spot: The area in the visual field that corresponds to the lack of photoreceptors at the optic disc.

Cataract: Clouding of the lens inside the eye, leading to a decrease in vision.

Confrontation visual field testing: A basic method to screen for visual field defects.

Corneal topography: A diagnostic tool that maps the curvature of the cornea.

Diabetic retinopathy: Damage to the retina caused by complications of diabetes, which can lead to blindness.

Direct ophthalmoscopy: A technique to view the interior surface of the eye, including the retina.

Electroretinography: A test that measures the electrical responses of the retina's light-sensitive cells (rods and cones).

External examination: Inspection of the eyelids, eyelashes and surrounding tissues for abnormalities.

Fluorescein angiography: A technique for examining blood circulation in the retina and choroid using a fluorescent dye.

Fundus photography: Capturing detailed images of the retina, optic disc and macula.

Gonioscopy: A diagnostic procedure to examine the anterior chamber angle of the eye.

Glaucoma: A group of eye conditions that damage the optic nerve, often associated with high intraocular pressure.

Indirect ophthalmoscopy: A method that provides a wide field of view of the retina using a condensing lens and a light source.

Intraocular pressure: The fluid pressure inside the eye.

Macular degeneration: An age-related condition that affects the central part of the retina (macula), leading to loss of central vision.

Macula: The central part of the retina responsible for detailed vision.

Ophthalmoscope: An instrument used to examine the interior of the eye.

Optical coherence tomography: A non-invasive imaging test that provides high-resolution cross-sectional images of the retina.

Optic disc: The point in the eye where the optic nerve fibres leave the retina.

Pachymetry: Measurement of corneal thickness.

Peripheral vision: The part of vision that occurs outside the very centre of gaze.

Photophobia: Sensitivity to light.

Pupil examination: Assessment of the pupil's size, shape and reactivity to light.

Retina: The light-sensitive layer at the back of the eye that converts light into neural signals.

Retinal detachment: A condition where the retina peels away from its underlying layer of support tissue.

Tonometry: A test to measure the pressure inside the eye.

Visual acuity: Sharpness or clarity of vision, typically measured with a Snellen chart.

Visual field: The entire area that can be seen when the eye is directed forward, including peripheral vision.

MULTIPLE CHOICE QUESTIONS

1. What is the first step in a comprehensive eye examination?
   a) Visual acuity test
   b) Pupillary examination
   c) External inspection of the eye
   d) Taking patient history

2. What is the purpose of fluorescein dye in an eye examination?
   a) To measure intraocular pressure
   b) To highlight scratches or abrasions on the cornea
   c) To test for colour vision defects
   d) To dilate the pupils

3. What should be avoided if a patient has a suspected penetrating eye injury?
   a) Using a slit lamp
   b) Instilling local anaesthetic drops
   c) Performing a pupillary light reflex test
   d) Using fluorescein dye

4. Which test is used to measure visual acuity?
   a) Snellen chart
   b) Amsler grid
   c) Tonometry
   d) Fundus photography

5. What is the function of the corneal topography test?
   a) To measure intraocular pressure
   b) To map the curvature of the cornea
   c) To examine the optic nerve head
   d) To evaluate the macula

6. Which reflex is checked to evaluate the integrity of the optic and oculomotor nerves?
   a) Blink reflex
   b) Pupillary light reflex
   c) Accommodation reflex
   d) Corneal reflex

7. What is the main purpose of measuring intraocular pressure (IOP)?
   a) To diagnose cataracts
   b) To screen for glaucoma
   c) To assess retinal health
   d) To evaluate macular function

8. Which structure is primarily examined using an ophthalmoscope?
   a) Cornea
   b) Retina
   c) Lens
   d) Iris

9. What is the purpose of the Amsler grid test?
   a) To measure intraocular pressure
   b) To assess central visual field
   c) To test for colour blindness
   d) To evaluate tear production

10. What is ptosis?
    a) Inflammation of the conjunctiva
    b) Drooping of the upper eyelid
    c) Blurring of vision
    d) Swelling of the cornea

REFERENCES

Borooah, S. and Tint, N.L. (2023). The visual system (Chapter 8). In: *Macleod's Clinical Examination*, 15e (eds. A.R. Dover, J.A. Innes, and K. Fairhurst). London: Elsevier.

Galloway, N.R., Amoaku, W.M., Galloway, P.H. et al. (2022). *Common Eye Diseases and their Management*, 5e. London: Springer.

Gibbons, H. (2019). Examinations of the eye (Chapter 11). In: *Physical Assessment for Nurses and Healthcare Professionals*, 3e (ed. C.L. Cox). Oxford: Wiley.

Jarvis, C. and Eckhradt, A. (2024). *Physical Examination and Health Assessment*, 9e. St Louis: Elsevier.

Meakin, S. and Seewoodhary, M. (2022). The person with an ear or eye disorder (Chapter 33). In: *Nursing Practice*, 3e (eds. I. Peate and A. Mitchell). Oxford: Wiley.

Needham, Y. (2019). Ophthalmological disorders (Chapter 3). In: *Learning to Care* (ed. I. Peate). London: Elsevier.

O'Driscoll, S. (2022). Neurological critical care (Chapter 14). In: *Fundamentals of Critical Care* (eds. I. Peate and B. Hill). Oxford: Wiley.

Phillips, A. (2023). *Diabetes Care at a Glance*. Oxford: Wiley.

Rhoads, J. and Wiggins Petersen, S. (2021). *Advanced Health Assessment and Diagnostic Reasoning*, 4e. Burlington: Jones and Bartlett.

Royal College of Ophthalmologists (2015). Snellen and LogMAR acuity testing. https://curriculum.rcophth.ac.uk/wp-content/uploads/2015/11/LogMAR-vs-Snellen.pdf (accessed July 2024).

Royal National Institute of Blind People (2021). Key statistics about sight loss. https://media.rnib.org.uk/documents/Key_stats_about_sight_loss_2021.pdf (accessed July 2024).

Sanderson, A. (2019). Nursing patients with disorders of the eye and sight impairment (Chapter 14). In: *Alexander's Nursing Practice*, 5e (ed. I. Peate). London: Elsevier.

The word glaucoma originates from the Greek word 'glaukos', which means 'shining' or 'bluish-green'. In ancient Greek, the term 'glaukos' was often used to describe the colour of the sea or the eyes of certain animals. In the context of healthcare, it referred to a condition of the eye characterised by a bluish-green appearance of the pupil due to clouding of the cornea or increased intraocular pressure (IOP), which are symptoms associated with the disease known as glaucoma. The term was later adopted into Latin as 'glaucoma' and then into English with the same spelling.

Glaucoma is a group of eye diseases that can cause irreversible loss of vision. The term is applied to a group of conditions that result in damage to the neural tissue of the retina and the optic nerve (Sanderson 2019). The diseases are quite distinct, and the treatment in each case is quite different. Glaucoma might be defined as a 'pathological level of IOP sufficient to damage vision'. This is to distinguish the normal elevation of IOP seen in otherwise normal individuals (Galloway et al. 2022). There are several types of glaucoma, each with distinct characteristics (see Table 3.1).

Each type of glaucoma identified in Table 3.1 requires specific diagnosis and treatment to manage and prevent vision loss. Regular eye examinations are crucial for early detection and management of this disease.

This chapter focuses predominantly on primary open-angle glaucoma (open-angle glaucoma).

PATHOPHYSIOLOGICAL CHANGES ASSOCIATED WITH PRIMARY OPEN-ANGLE GLAUCOMA

RAISED INTRAOCULAR PRESSURE

Intraocular pressure refers to the fluid pressure inside the eye. It plays an essential role in maintaining the eye's shape and its proper functioning. IOP is measured during eye examinations to assess eye health and to detect conditions such as glaucoma. The average normal IOP ranges between 10 and 21 mmHg (Vaz, Mehta, and Hamilton 2021). If IOP remains too high or too low, it can impact vision and eye health. The National Institute for Health and Care Excellence [NICE] (2022) notes that an upper level of 21 mmHg is often accepted, when pressure rises above this level, suspicions are raised and there is a need for further investigations to be undertaken. Some types of glaucoma can reach pressures exceeding 70 mmHg (Vaz, Mehta, and Hamilton 2021).

MAINTAINING INTRAOCULAR PRESSURE

If the eye is to function as an effective optical instrument, IOP must be maintained at a constant level. At the same time, active circulation of fluid through the globe is essential if the structures within it are to receive adequate nourishment. The cornea and sclera form a tough, fibrous and unyielding envelope and within this an even pressure is maintained by a balance between the production and drainage of aqueous fluid.

Table 3.1 Types of glaucoma

Type of glaucoma	Characteristics
Primary open-angle glaucoma	This is the most common type of glaucoma. It develops slowly and painlessly, often without noticeable symptoms, until significant vision loss has occurred. The drainage canals in the eye become blocked over time, leading to increased eye pressure.
Angle-closure glaucoma	Also known as closed-angle glaucoma or narrow-angle glaucoma. This type of glaucoma can be chronic or acute. The condition occurs when the iris bulges forward to narrow or block the drainage angle formed by the cornea and iris, leading to a sudden increase in intraocular pressure (IOP). Symptoms of acute angle-closure glaucoma include severe eye pain, nausea, redness and blurred vision.
Normal-tension glaucoma	Also known as low-tension or normal-pressure glaucoma. The optic nerve is damaged even though the IOP is within the normal range. The exact cause is unknown, but it may be related to a sensitive optic nerve or reduced blood flow to the optic nerve.
Secondary glaucoma	Secondary glaucoma results from another medical condition, such as inflammation, trauma or diabetes, which increases the IOP. The types include: • Pigmentary glaucoma: caused by pigment granules from the iris that block the drainage canals. • Neovascular glaucoma: associated with abnormal blood vessel growth that blocks the eye's drainage channels. • Exfoliative glaucoma: characterised by a flaky, dandruff-like material that peels off the outer layer of the lens and blocks the drainage system. • Traumatic glaucoma: resulting from an eye injury.
Congenital glaucoma	Present at birth. Caused by an abnormal development of the eye's drainage system during the prenatal period. Symptoms include enlarged eyes, cloudiness (the cornea, the clear front part of the eye, may become cloudy or hazy due to oedema [swelling] or damage from increased pressure) and sensitivity to light.
Juvenile glaucoma	Occurs in children, adolescents and young adults. Usually this is inherited, and it often results in a more severe and rapid increase in eye pressure.

Source: Adapted from Sanderson (2019); Galloway et al. (2022).

Aqueous humour is produced by the ciliary epithelium by active secretion and ultrafiltration. Ultrafiltration is the passive movement of water and small molecules from the blood vessels into the eye due to pressure differences. This process filters out larger molecules and cells, allowing only water and small solutes to pass through, contributing to the formation of the aqueous humour. A continuous flow is maintained through the pupil, where it reaches the angle of the anterior chamber. On reaching the angle of the anterior chamber, the aqueous humour passes through the trabecular meshwork and then reaches a circular canal embedded in the sclera known as Schlemm's canal (Huether and Rodway 2019). Schlemm's canal acts as a ring that collects aqueous humour and then tiny channels carry this fluid to veins outside the eye for drainage. These channels are known as aqueous veins and they transmit clear aqueous to the episcleral veins, which lie in the connective tissue underlying the conjunctiva.

Although it is known that the ciliary epithelium produces aqueous humour and the trabecular meshwork helps drain it, the exact roles and how they work together to keep the eye pressure stable over a person's lifetime are not completely understood. While the eye actively produces aqueous humour, it drains out more naturally. Adjusting the muscle that affects fluid flow can impact how quickly the fluid leaves the eye and its rate of drainage.

Intraocular pressure naturally changes throughout the day. It tends to be at its highest level in the early morning and usually decreases as the day progresses. If the normal daily fluctuation in IOP becomes more extreme, this might be an early sign of glaucoma (Galloway et al. 2022).

The optic nerve carries visual information from the eye to the brain through the axons of retinal ganglion cells. When these nerve fibres are damaged, it can lead to the death of ganglion cells, causing optic nerve atrophy and patchy vision loss (Huether and Rodway 2019). Elevated IOP can contribute to this damage, either by directly compressing the nerve or reducing blood flow to it. However, the relationship between IOP and nerve damage is complex.

Externally measured IOP might not always reflect the true pressure inside the eye. Variations in corneal thickness can lead to inaccurate IOP readings as thinner corneas can make the pressure seem higher, while thicker corneas can make it seem lower. Additionally, issues with blood flow to the optic nerve and factors within the optic nerve itself may influence its susceptibility to damage.

Intraocular pressure is regulated by the balance between the production and drainage of aqueous humour. Elevated IOP usually occurs because of problems with fluid drainage rather than excessive fluid production. In open-angle glaucoma, the drainage system appears clear, but the outflow is insufficient (see Figure 3.1). In angle-closure glaucoma, the drainage is physically blocked by the iris, leading to increased pressure.

EPIDEMIOLOGY

Glaucoma is a significant public health issue. Globally, glaucoma is the second most common cause of blindness. In the UK, it is the most common cause of blind registration (Vaz, Mehta, and Hamilton 2021; Royal National Institute of Blind People 2021). Glaucoma is one of the most common eye conditions encountered in primary and secondary care. Worldwide, glaucoma accounted for 7.7 million people with moderate or severe visual impairment in 2020 (World Health Organization 2023). The most common overall cause was cataract (88.4 million; Global Burden of Disease Study 2019). The social burden and economic burden of glaucoma are likely to increase in the future because of longer life expectancy and an ageing population.

Glaucoma-related hospital outpatient visits in England exceed one million annually. This high number reflects the ongoing management and treatment needs of patients with glaucoma (Fu et al. 2023). It is estimated that about 2% of people aged 40 years plus have

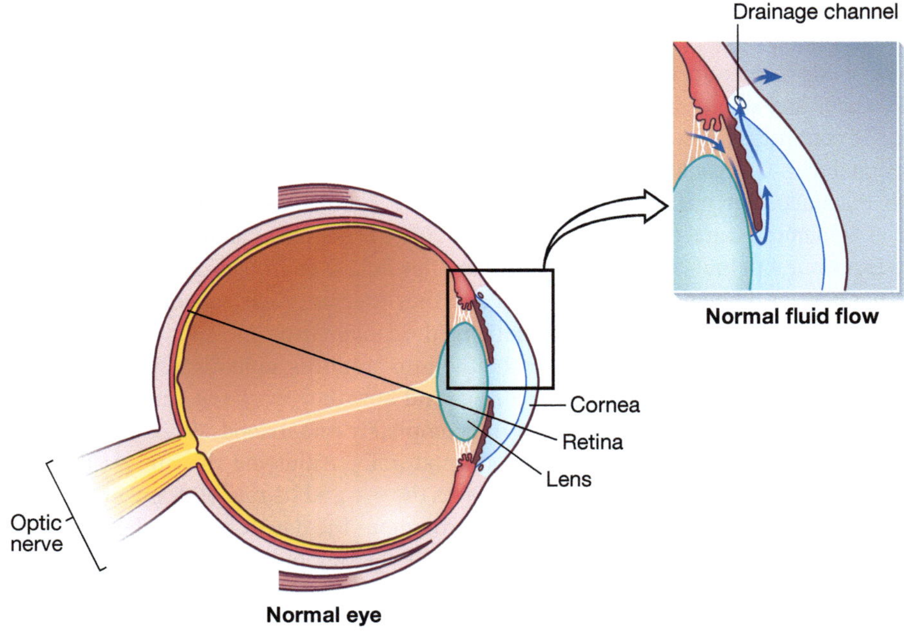

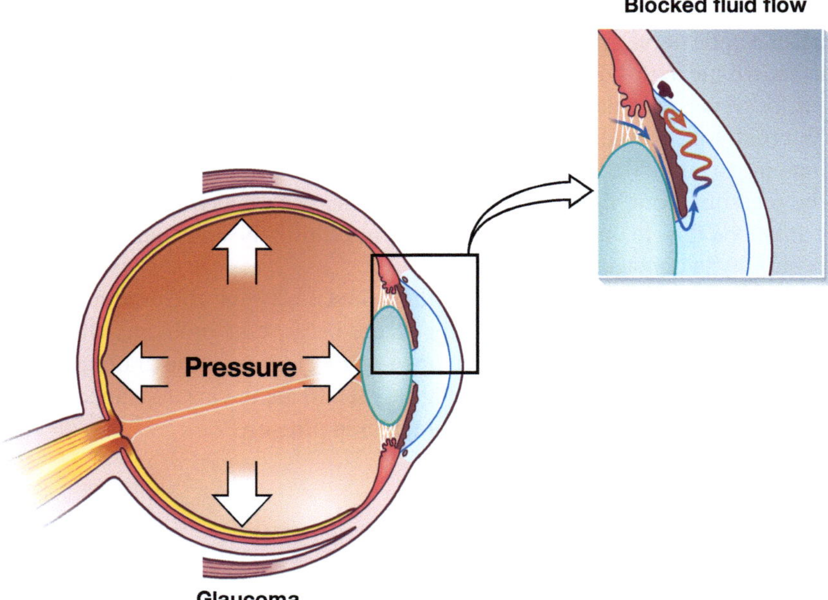

FIGURE 3.1 Glaucoma

primary open-angle glaucoma and this rises to almost 10% in people older than 75 years (Glaucoma UK 2020).

Certain ethnic groups, particularly those of African or Caribbean descent, are at higher risk for developing glaucoma. Research shows that these groups have a higher incidence and a greater risk of more severe forms of the disease (Nagar et al. 2020).

RISK FACTORS

Glaucoma is a complex eye condition with various risk factors that can contribute to its development. Understanding these risk factors can aid in early detection and management. The main risk factors associated with glaucoma are provided in Table 3.2.

Table 3.2   Key risk factors associated with glaucoma

Risk factor	Discussion
Age	Increased risk with age: The risk of developing glaucoma increases significantly with age. People over 60 years are at higher risk, with the prevalence increasing to about 10% in those over 75 years old.
Family history	Genetic redisposition: A family history of glaucoma increases an individual's risk. First-degree relatives of glaucoma patients are at a significantly higher risk due to genetic factors.
Ethnicity	Higher risk in certain ethnic groups: People of African, Caribbean or Hispanic descent have a higher risk of developing glaucoma. These populations also tend to develop the condition at an earlier age and are more likely to experience severe vision loss. Asian descent: Individuals of Asian descent are at increased risk for angle-closure glaucoma.
Elevated intraocular pressure (IOP)	Primary risk factor: High IOP is the most significant risk factor for glaucoma. However, it is worth noting that some people with normal IOP can still develop glaucoma (normal-tension glaucoma) and not everyone with high IOP will develop the condition (ocular hypertension).
Medical conditions	Diabetes: Individuals with diabetes are at an increased risk of developing glaucoma. Hypertension: High blood pressure is another contributing factor. Cardiovascular disease: Certain heart conditions and other vascular diseases can increase the risk.
Eye conditions and injuries	Previous eye injuries: Trauma to the eye can lead to secondary glaucoma. Other eye conditions: Conditions such as severe myopia (near-sightedness), retinal detachment and chronic eye inflammation (uveitis) can increase glaucoma risk.
Use of corticosteroids	Long-term use: Prolonged use of corticosteroid medications, whether oral, topical or inhaled, can increase the risk of developing glaucoma.
Thin corneas	Corneal thickness: A thinner central cornea is a risk factor for developing glaucoma, as it can lead to underestimated IOP readings and may indicate structural weaknesses in the eye.
Lifestyle factors	Smoking: Smoking has been linked to an increased risk of glaucoma. Poor diet: Diets lacking in essential nutrients that support eye health may contribute to the development of glaucoma.
Low blood pressure	Hypotension: Low blood pressure can reduce the blood flow to the optic nerve, increasing the risk of damage.

Source: King, Azuara-Blanco, and Tuulonen (2013), National Eye Institute (2021) and American Optometric Association (2024).

Glaucoma is influenced by a variety of risk factors, including age, family history, ethnicity, elevated IOP, medical conditions, eye injuries, use of corticosteroids, corneal thickness, lifestyle factors and hypotension. Recognising these risk factors is essential for early detection and effective management of glaucoma to prevent vision loss.

CLINICAL PRESENTATION

Huether and Rodway (2019) note that extremely high IOP can cause blindness within days or hours. Most patients with chronic glaucoma do not experience any symptoms; the disease progresses slowly and is often only detected during a routine eye examination by an optometrist or ophthalmologist, before the patient notices any visual loss. Unfortunately, the peripheral loss of vision can go unnoticed until it reaches an advanced stage. Symptoms of primary open-angle glaucoma are usually asymptomatic until there is significant loss of visual field. Galloway et al. (2022) report that there are three cardinal signs associated with glaucoma:

1. Raised IOP
2. Cupping of the optic disc
3. Visual field loss

RAISED INTRAOCULAR PRESSURE

Intraocular pressure is the fluid pressure inside the eye. This occurs when the aqueous humour (the clear fluid inside the eye) is produced faster than it can drain out. This imbalance leads to increased pressure within the eye. High IOP is a significant finding/risk factor for glaucoma because it can damage the optic nerve, which is essential for vision. Elevated IOP alone does not mean a person has glaucoma, but it increases the risk.

CUPPING OF THE OPTIC DISC

The optic disc is the region at the back of the eye where the optic nerve fibres exit the retina. Cupping refers to a hollowed-out appearance of the optic disc. Raised IOP can damage the optic nerve fibres, leading to the loss of these fibres and the subsequent appearance of cupping. Optic disc cupping is a hallmark of glaucomatous damage. The cup-to-disc ratio is used to describe the extent of cupping.

The cup-to-disc ratio is a critical metric used to assess the health of the optic nerve and to identify potential damage caused by glaucoma. It provides a way to quantify the extent of cupping in the optic disc, with higher ratios indicating more significant cupping and potential optic nerve damage. Regular monitoring of this ratio helps in early detection and management of glaucoma to prevent vision loss. Progressive cupping suggests worsening glaucoma.

VISUAL FIELD LOSS

This refers to the loss of peripheral vision that can progress to affect central vision if glaucoma remains untreated. Visual field loss is typically detected through visual field tests, such as perimetry. These tests map out the patient's field of vision and identify areas of lost or reduced vision. Early-stage glaucoma often has no noticeable symptoms. As the disease progresses, patients may begin to notice 'blind spots' in their peripheral vision. In advanced stages, vision loss can become more significant and affect central vision. Glaucomatous visual field loss often starts in an arcuate (arc-shaped) pattern around the central vision. As the damage progresses, these areas can enlarge and coalesce, leading to significant peripheral vision loss.

CLINICAL INVESTIGATIONS AND DIAGNOSIS

The onset of open-angle glaucoma is gradual, often leaving patients unaware of their condition. Despite maintaining good visual acuity, they may have severe disease. Those with more advanced stages may notice shadows in their vision or a reduction in visual acuity. A normal visual field in one eye can obscure a defect in the affected eye until the disease is significantly progressed. Diagnosing this silent disease is crucial. When a diagnosis is missed, it can result in losing the opportunity to stop its progression, while misdiagnosis can lead to unnecessary lifelong medication (Galloway et al. 2022).

Patients suspected of having glaucoma require a thorough ocular examination to rule out coexisting conditions or other diagnoses. The assessment process has to be systematic and comprehensive. A detailed history is taken and the eye is examined thoroughly for evidence of glaucoma, comorbidity or an alternative diagnosis to the apparent findings. Local policy and procedure must be adhered to regarding the use of a chaperone, consent and infection control and prevention.

PATIENT HISTORY

Performing a medical history review for glaucoma involves a detailed and structured interview process. The following steps are usually undertaken in conducting a medical history review for glaucoma.

Initial Patient Interview   Introductions and explanations underpinning the interview are undertaken with an emphasis on the importance of gathering accurate information for a comprehensive glaucoma assessment.

Medical History   Inquiries are made about the patient's overall health and any chronic conditions such as diabetes, hypertension and migraines. The patient is asked about any past eye conditions (e.g. ocular hypertension, previous eye injuries or surgery) and treatments. A review of all current and past medications, especially corticosteroids, which can elevate IOP, is undertaken. Any current or past symptoms related to vision, such as blurred vision, halos around lights, eye pain, headaches or any changes in visual field, are addressed.

FAMILY HISTORY

The patient is asked if any close family members, particularly parents or siblings, have been diagnosed with glaucoma or had eye diseases. Inquiries are made about other hereditary conditions that may affect eye health.

DISCUSSIONS REGARDING RISK FACTORS

Document the patient's age, noting that the risk of glaucoma increases significantly after the age of 40 years. Record the patient's ethnicity, as certain ethnic groups have higher risks for specific types of glaucoma. The patient is specifically asked about conditions such as diabetes, hypertension and hypotension that can influence glaucoma risk. The person is asked about corticosteroid use, the duration, dosage and type of corticosteroid used.

LIFESTYLE AND ENVIRONMENTAL FACTORS

Assessment is made to determine if the patient's job involves activities that might affect eye health, such as exposure to chemicals or prolonged use of visual display units. Inquiries are made about smoking or alcohol consumption, which may impact overall health and eye health indirectly.

Review of previous eye examinations and their outcomes is important. If possible, records are reviewed from previous eye examinations to note any changes in IOP, optic nerve condition or visual field tests. A baseline is provided for future comparisons, especially if there is a history of elevated intraocular or optic nerve changes.

Performing a medical history review for glaucoma involves a detailed interview process where information is gathered about the patient's general health, specific eye health, family history and lifestyle factors. This review helps identify risk factors, guide further testing and tailor the management plan for glaucoma, aiming for early detection and effective treatment to prevent vision loss.

EXAMINATION AND INVESTIGATIONS

Guidance issued by NICE (2022) notes that prior to referral for glaucoma assessment, the following are required:

- Gonioscopy, a technique used to measure the angle between the cornea and the iris to assess whether the glaucoma is open-angle or closed-angle. A mirror is placed on the surface of the numbed eye, which allows direct measurement of the angle.

- Corneal thickness assessment: Corneal thickness influences the IOP reading. If it is thicker than usual, it will take greater force to indent the cornea and an erroneously high reading will be obtained (this is also true for a thin cornea). Corneal thickness is measured by pachymetry.

- Tonometry optic disc examination permits the objective measurement of IOP, usually based on the assessment of resistance of the cornea to indent.

- Optic disc examination: This provides a direct marker for disease progression. Optic disc damage is assessed by looking at the ratio of the diameters of the pale centre (cup) to the overall size of the disc. The normal cup-to-disc ratio is 0.3, although it can be up to 0.7 in some people without glaucoma.

- Visual fields are assessed. Assessing visual fields includes the use of perimetry, which objectively documents what the patient perceives in the periphery of their vision. These assessments can be affected by fatigue, spectacle frames, miosis, media opacities, as well as cooperation of the patient.

MANAGEMENT

Management of glaucoma can vary widely among healthcare providers. National guidelines, such as those from NICE (2022), offer standardised recommendations. Treatment may not start immediately because multiple assessments are needed to confirm the diagnosis, given the potential for variable findings. Glaucoma is a significant condition requiring lifelong treatment. In cases where the disease is clearly advanced, treatment should begin without delay to prevent further vision loss.

Balancing the most effective treatment with the individual's needs is essential. Making treatment decisions in partnership with the individual fosters ownership and supports adherence to treatment regimens. Therefore, it is essential to listen to and record any concerns. Often, during vision tests, patients will share how they feel and how they are coping. Providing advice about support and where to access it is important, such as directing patients to the International Glaucoma Association and Royal National Institute of Blind People, especially if they have registrable visual loss (Needham 2019). The fear of sight loss can lead to depression, particularly in older adults, as it can impact all aspects of life. Offering practical and emotional support can boost confidence and help individuals live with this long-term condition. Three approaches to management are available.

- Laser surgery

- Incisional surgery

- Medications

The type of glaucoma determines the appropriate method or methods. The three approaches are discussed in Table 3.3.

Table 3.3   Approaches to the management of glaucoma

Approach	Advantages	Disadvantages
Laser surgery Laser surgery involves using focused light energy to treat the trabecular meshwork, the part of the eye responsible for draining aqueous humour or to create a new drainage pathway. Types of laser surgery: Selective laser trabeculoplasty (SLT): This procedure uses low-energy laser pulses to target specific cells in the trabecular meshwork, improving aqueous outflow. It is often used as an initial treatment or when medications fail. Argon laser trabeculoplasty: Similar to SLT but uses a different type of laser. It also aims to improve drainage through the trabecular meshwork but can cause more thermal damage than SLT. Laser peripheral iridotomy: Primarily used for angle-closure glaucoma, this procedure creates a small hole in the iris to allow aqueous humour to flow more freely within the eye. Cyclophotocoagulation: This procedure targets the ciliary body, reducing the production of aqueous humour and lowering IOP.	Minimally invasive Outpatient procedure with quick recovery Effective for many patients, either as a primary treatment or adjunct to medications	Effect may diminish over time Potential for complications, such as inflammation or increased intraocular pressure (IOP) shortly after the procedure

(Continued)

Table 3.3 (*Continued*)

Approach	Advantages	Disadvantages
Incisional surgery Incisional surgery, also known as filtering surgery, involves making incisions in the eye to create a new pathway for aqueous humour drainage. Types of incisional surgery: Trabeculectomy: The most common glaucoma surgery, where a small piece of the trabecular meshwork is removed to create a new drainage channel. Aqueous humour drains into a bleb (a small blister-like area) formed under the conjunctiva, where it is absorbed. Glaucoma drainage devices: Also known as shunts or tubes, these devices are implanted in the eye to facilitate aqueous drainage. Examples include the Ahmed valve and Baerveldt implant. Minimally invasive glaucoma surgery: These newer techniques involve smaller incisions and devices, such as the iStent, Hydrus Microstent and Trabectome, to enhance aqueous outflow with less tissue damage and quicker recovery.	Can significantly lower IOP, especially in advanced cases Effective when medications and laser treatments are insufficient	More invasive with longer recovery times Higher risk of complications, such as infection, bleeding and scarring
Medications Medications are typically the first line of treatment for glaucoma and aim to either decrease the production of aqueous humour or increase its outflow. Types of medications: Prostaglandins: Increase outflow of aqueous humour (such as latanoprost, travoprost, bimatoprost). Beta blockers: Reduce aqueous humour production (i.e. timolol, betaxolol, levubunolol, carteolol). Alpha agonists: Decrease production and increase outflow of aqueous humour (brimonidine, apraclonidine). Carbonic anhydrase inhibitors: Reduce aqueous humour production (dorzolamide, brinzolamide). Combination drugs: Combine two or more types of medication to increase effectiveness and improve adherence (e.g. timolol and dorzolamide).	Non-invasive Easy to administer (usually in the form of eye drops) Can be tailored to individual patient needs	Potential side effects, such as redness, stinging or systemic effects (e.g. heart rate changes with beta blockers) Adherence can be a challenge, especially with multiple medications or frequent dosing

Source: Adapted from Galloway et al. (2022); NICE (2022).

In summary, the management of glaucoma can be approached through laser surgery, incisional surgery and medications. Each approach has its benefits and drawbacks and the choice of treatment depends on the severity of the disease, patient preferences and response to previous treatments. Laser surgery is less invasive and can be effective as a primary treatment or adjunct. Incisional surgery is more invasive but necessary for advanced cases. Medications are typically the first line of treatment and are effective in many cases but require patient adherence and can have side effects.

HEALTH TEACHING

Addressing the health teaching needs for people with glaucoma is important for effective management of the condition and preventing further vision loss. It involves providing information to patients about their disease, treatment options, lifestyle adjustments and the importance of concordance with prescribed medication regimens. The key aspects that should be considered in relation to the health teaching needs of people with glaucoma include the following:

DISEASE EXPLANATION

Inform patients about what glaucoma is, including its causes, risk factors and how it damages the optic nerve, leading to vision loss. Explain the different types of glaucoma (e.g. primary open-angle glaucoma, angle-closure glaucoma) and how they differ in terms of symptoms and treatment.

SYMPTOMS AWARENESS

Explain to patients that glaucoma often has no early symptoms and that vision loss typically starts peripherally and progresses without noticeable signs until advanced stages. Encourage patients to report any changes in vision, eye pain or other unusual symptoms immediately.

TREATMENT ADHERENCE

Explain to the patient the importance of taking prescribed medications regularly, as missing doses can lead to increased IOP and further optic nerve damage. Provide clear instructions on how to use eye drops correctly, including tips for ensuring the medication is properly administered. See also Box 3.1.

APPOINTMENT KEEPING

Stress the necessity of regular follow-up visits for monitoring IOP, assessing the effectiveness of treatments and making necessary adjustments. Advise on the frequency of these visits, which can vary based on the stage and severity of glaucoma.

LIFESTYLE ADJUSTMENTS

Recommend protective eyewear to prevent injuries that could exacerbate glaucoma. Suggest avoiding activities that can increase IOP, such as heavy lifting or straining.

Encourage a balanced diet rich in antioxidants, vitamins and minerals that support eye health. Advocate for regular exercise, which can help lower IOP, but advise avoiding exercises that involve head-down positions.

In the UK, glaucoma can affect a person's ability to drive due to the disease's impact on peripheral vision. The Driving Vehicle and Licencing Agency requires individuals diagnosed with glaucoma in both eyes to report their condition and undergo assessments to determine if they meet the visual standards for driving. Failure to meet these standards can result in the withdrawal of their driving licence. Support and resources are available to help individuals navigate the implications of glaucoma on their driving abilities and maintain their independence where possible.

EMOTIONAL SUPPORT

Discuss the emotional impact of glaucoma, including fear of blindness and potential depression. Provide reassurance and realistic expectations about disease progression and treatment outcomes. Inform patients about support groups and counselling services, which can provide emotional support and practical advice from others with glaucoma. Recommend resources such as the International Glaucoma Association and the Royal National Institute of Blind People for additional support and information.

EMERGENCY SITUATIONS

Provide the patient with information on recognising signs of acute glaucoma attacks, such as sudden eye pain, headache, nausea and blurred vision and the need for immediate medical attention.

Poor compliance with medication is common amongst some people with glaucoma (Chung 2020). Encouraging patients to adhere to their eye drop regimen for glaucoma treatment involves a multifaceted approach. Box 3.1 identifies some strategies that may help.

BOX 3.1   **APPROACHES TO IMPROVING MEDICATION CONCORDANCE**

Information and communication

Informative sessions: Provide detailed information about glaucoma, the importance of eye drops in preventing vision loss and the consequences of non-adherence.

1. Clear instructions: Ensure patients understand how to correctly use their eye drops, including the correct dosage, timing and storage.

2. Written materials: Offer brochures or leaflets alongside step-by-step instructions and information about glaucoma.

3. Demonstrations: Demonstrate the correct way to administer the eye drops during consultations.

Reminders and follow-ups

1. Reminders: Use phone calls, text messages or apps to remind patients to take their medication.

2. Appointment scheduling: Schedule regular follow-up appointments to monitor adherence and address any issues.

3. Personalised follow-up: Contact patients who miss appointments or report difficulties to provide additional support.

Simplifying the regimen

1. Once-daily dosing: When possible, eye drops should be prescribed that require less frequent dosing.

2. Combining medications: Use combination eye drops to reduce the number of administrations per day.

3. Convenient packaging: Ensure the eye drop packaging is easy to open and handle, especially those who may have manual dexterity problems.

Addressing barriers

1. Side effects: Discuss potential side effects and manage them proactively to improve comfort and adherence.

2. Access: Help patients obtain their medication regularly by coordinating with pharmacies or arranging delivery services.

Building a support system

1. Family involvement: If appropriate, encourage family members to support the patient in managing their treatment.

2. Support groups: Recommend support groups where patients can share experiences and tips for adherence.

Motivational strategies

1. Positive reinforcement: Emphasise positive outcomes.

2. Setting goals: Work with patients to set realistic adherence goals and track progress.

3. Self-monitoring: Encourage patients to keep a diary or use an app to record their eye drop usage.

Professional support

1. Regular check-ins: Offer regular check-ins to provide support and answer questions.

2. Tailored interventions: Develop personalised interventions based on individual patient needs and challenges.

By combining education, reminders, support systems and motivational strategies, this can significantly improve adherence to eye drop regimens in patients with glaucoma.

Source: Glaucoma UK (2020); Needham (2019).

People should be offered the opportunity to discuss their diagnosis, referral, prognosis, treatment and discharge so they can take an active part in decision-making and this includes their use of medication. Provide the patient with relevant information in an accessible format at initial and subsequent visits. This entails telling them about the different types of treatment options, including mode of action, frequency and severity of side effects and risks and benefits of treatment (Sanderson 2019; Needham 2019).

CONCLUSION

Glaucoma represents a significant public health challenge due to its potential to cause irreversible vision loss and blindness if left untreated. This group of eye diseases is characterised by damage to the optic nerve, primarily associated with elevated IOP. The silent, progressive nature of glaucoma often leads to delayed diagnosis, emphasising the critical importance of regular eye examinations, particularly for high-risk populations.

Management of glaucoma involves a multifaceted approach, including medications, laser treatments and surgical interventions, aimed at reducing IOP to prevent further optic nerve damage. The choice of treatment is tailored to the individual patient, considering the type and severity of glaucoma, as well as the patient's overall health and lifestyle.

Patient education and adherence to treatment regimens are paramount. Health teaching needs to focus on ensuring patients understand the chronic nature of glaucoma, the importance of consistent medication use and the necessity of regular follow-up visits. Emotional and psychological support should also be provided to help patients cope with the potential fear and anxiety associated with vision loss.

GLOSSARY OF TERMS

Aqueous humour: The clear fluid produced by the ciliary body in the eye, filling the space between the cornea and the lens. It helps maintain intraocular pressure and provides nutrients to the avascular structures of the eye.

Angle-closure glaucoma: A type of glaucoma where the drainage angle formed by the cornea and the iris is blocked, leading to a rapid increase in intraocular pressure. It can cause sudden vision loss and is considered a medical emergency.

Ciliary body: The part of the eye that produces aqueous humour and contains the ciliary muscle, which controls the shape of the lens for focusing.

Cup-to-disc ratio: A measurement used to assess the optic nerve head for glaucoma. It compares the diameter of the optic cup to the diameter of the optic disc. An increased ratio may indicate glaucomatous damage.

Diurnal variation: The natural fluctuation of intraocular pressure throughout the day, typically highest in the early morning and decreasing throughout the day.

Glaucoma: A group of eye diseases characterised by damage to the optic nerve, often associated with elevated intraocular pressure, leading to progressive vision loss.

Intraocular pressure: The fluid pressure inside the eye. Maintaining a normal intraocular is crucial for the health of the optic nerve and overall eye function.

Laser surgery: A treatment method for glaucoma that uses focused light energy to improve aqueous humour outflow or reduce its production, thereby lowering intraocular pressure.

Optic nerve: The nerve that transmits visual information from the retina to the brain. Damage to the optic nerve in glaucoma can lead to vision loss.

Peripheral vision: The ability to see objects outside the direct line of sight. Glaucoma often affects peripheral vision first before impacting central vision.

Primary open-angle glaucoma (POAG): The most common form of glaucoma, characterised by a gradual increase in intraocular pressure due to reduced drainage of aqueous humour through the trabecular meshwork, with an open and unobstructed angle.

Selective laser trabeculoplasty: A laser surgery technique used to treat open-angle glaucoma by targeting specific cells in the trabecular meshwork to improve aqueous humour drainage.

Trabeculectomy: A surgical procedure to treat glaucoma by creating a new drainage pathway for aqueous humour to lower intraocular pressure.

Trabecular meshwork: The spongy tissue located near the base of the cornea, responsible for draining aqueous humour from the eye into Schlemm's canal.

Visual field test: A diagnostic test to assess a person's peripheral vision and detect any visual field loss, commonly used in glaucoma management.

Visual acuity: The clarity or sharpness of vision, usually measured with a Snellen chart. This is important in assessing overall eye health and the impact of glaucoma on vision.

MULTIPLE CHOICE QUESTIONS

1. What is the primary cause of vision loss in glaucoma?
   a) Cataracts
   b) Retinal detachment
   c) Optic nerve damage
   d) Macular degeneration

2. Which part of the eye is primarily responsible for producing aqueous humour?
   a) Retina
   b) Lens
   c) Ciliary body
   d) Optic nerve

3. What is the main function of the trabecular meshwork in the eye?
   a) Producing aqueous humour
   b) Draining aqueous humour
   c) Refracting light
   d) Supporting the lens

4. Which of the following is a common first-line medication for reducing intraocular pressure in glaucoma patients?
   a) Antibiotics
   b) Prostaglandin analogues
   c) Steroids
   d) Antihistamines

5. Which type of glaucoma occurs despite having normal intraocular pressure?
   a) Primary open-angle glaucoma
   b) Angle-closure glaucoma
   c) Normal-tension glaucoma
   d) Secondary glaucoma

6. What visual field defect is typically associated with glaucoma?
   a) Central vision loss
   b) Peripheral vision loss
   c) Colour vision loss
   d) Night vision loss

7. What surgical procedure creates a new drainage pathway for aqueous humour in glaucoma patients?
   a) Cataract surgery
   b) Trabeculectomy
   c) LASIK surgery
   d) Retinal detachment repair

8. Which laser treatment is commonly used for open-angle glaucoma to improve aqueous outflow?
   a) Photocoagulation
   b) Selective laser trabeculoplasty
   c) YAG capsulotomy
   d) Argon laser iridotomy

9. What is the cup-to-disc ratio used to assess?
   a) Corneal thickness
   b) Retinal detachment
   c) Optic nerve health
   d) Lens opacity

10. Which part of the eye does glaucoma primarily affect?
    a) Retina
    b) Cornea
    c) Optic nerve
    d) Iris

REFERENCES

American Optometric Association (2024). Glaucoma. https://www.aoa.org/healthy-eyes/eye-and-vision-conditions/glaucoma?sso=y (accessed July 2024).

Chung, S.Y. (2020). Addressing adherence in glaucoma patients, glaucoma today. https://assets.bmctoday.net/glaucomatoday/pdfs/0520GT_Residents%20&%20Fellows.pdf.

Fu, D.J., Ademisoye, E., Shih, V. et al. (2023). Burden of glaucoma in the United Kingdom. A multi-center analysis of United Kingdom glaucoma services. *Ophthalmol Glaucoma* 6 (1): 106–115. doi: 10.1016/j.ogla.2022.08.007.

Galloway, N.R., Amoaku, W.M., Galloway, P.H. et al. (2022). *Common Eye Diseases and Their Management*, 5e. London: Springer.

Glaucoma UK (2020). Eye drops and dispensing aids a guide. https://glaucoma.uk/wp-content/uploads/2020/07/3000_GlaucomaUK_PatientLeaflet_A5_EyeDropsandDispensingAids_Web.pdf (accessed July 2024).

Global Burden of Disease Study (2019). Blindness and Vision Impairment Collaborators; Vision Loss Expert Group of the Global Burden of Disease Study. Causes of blindness and vision impairment in 2020 and trends over 30 years, and prevalence of avoidable blindness in relation to vision 2020: the right to sight: an analysis for the global burden of disease study. *Lancet Global Health* 9 (2): e144–e160. doi: 10.1016/S2214-109X(20)30489-7.

Huether, S.E. and Rodway, E.W. (2019). Pain, temperature regulation, sleep and sensory function (Chapter 16). In: *Pathophysiology. The Biologic Basis for Disease in Adults and Children*, 8e (eds. K.L. McCance and S.E. Huether). St Louis: Elsevier.

King, A., Azuara-Blanco, A., and Tuulonen, A., (2013). Glaucoma. *British Medical Journal* 346. 3518, doi: 10.1136/bmj.f3518.

Nagar, A., Myeres, S., Kozareva, D. et al. (2020). Cascade screening for glaucoma in high-risk family members of African-Caribbean glaucoma patients in an urban population in London. *British Journal of Ophthalmology* 106 (3): 376–380. doi:10.1136/bjophthalmol-2020-317373.

National Eye Institute (2021). Types of glaucoma. https://www.aoa.org/healthy-eyes/eye-and-vision-conditions/glaucoma?sso=y (accessed July 2024).

National Institute for Health and Care Excellence (2022). Glaucoma: diagnosis and management. https://www.nice.org.uk/guidance/ng81/resources/glaucoma-diagnosis-and-management-pdf-1837689655237 (accessed July 2024).

Needham, Y. (2019). Ophthalmological disorders (Chapter 3). In: *Learning to Care* (ed. I. Peate). London: Elsevier.

Royal National Institute of Blind People (2021). Key statistics about sight loss. https://media.rnib.org.uk/documents/Key_stats_about_sight_loss_2021.pdf (accessed July 2024).

Sanderson, A. (2019). Nursing patients with disorders of the eye and sight impairment (Chapter 14). In: *Alexander's Nursing Practice*, 5e (ed. I. Peate). London: Elsevier.

Vaz, F., Mehta, N., and Hamilton, R.D. (2021). Ear, nose and throat and eye disease (Chapter 27). In: *Kumar and Clark's Clinical Medicine*, 10e (eds. A. Feather, D. Randall, and M. Waterhouse). London: Elsevier.

World Health Organization (2023). Blindness and vision impairment. https://www.who.int/news-room/fact-sheets/detail/blindness-and-visual-impairment (accessed July 2024).

The word 'cataract' originally comes from Latin and Greek. In Latin, 'cataracta' means 'waterfall' or a type of heavy door. This Latin word was borrowed from the Greek word 'kataraktes', which also means 'waterfall'. In Greek, 'kataraktes' combines 'kata', meaning 'down', and 'rheō', meaning 'to flow'. Accordingly, it literally means 'flowing down'.

In medicine, 'cataract' was chosen to describe a clouding of the lens in the eye. The reason is metaphorical: just as a waterfall blocks a clear view with its cascade, a cataract in the eye blocks clear vision because the lens becomes cloudy. The term helps illustrate how the lens, when affected by a cataract, obstructs light and vision, similar to how a waterfall can block what you see behind it. See Figures 4.1 and 4.2 a,b.

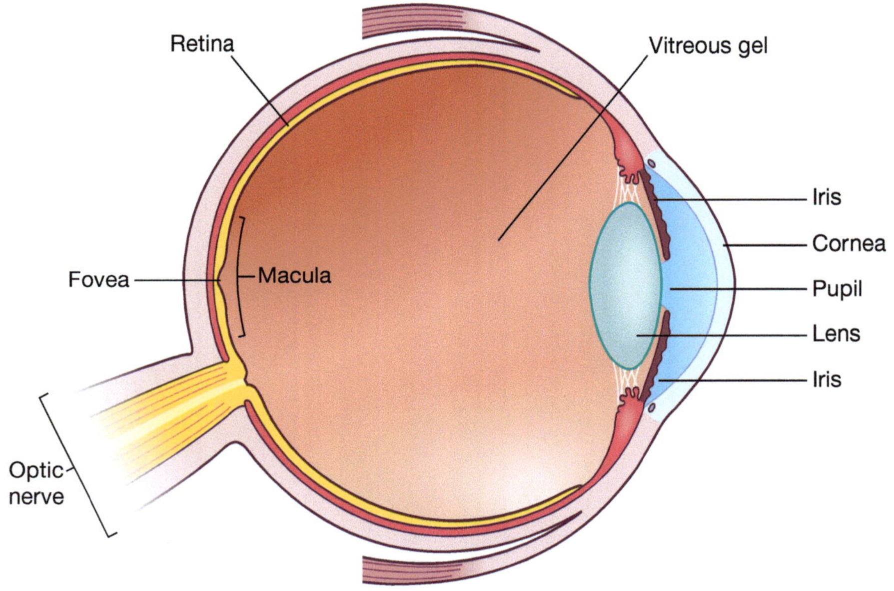

FIGURE 4.1 The eye

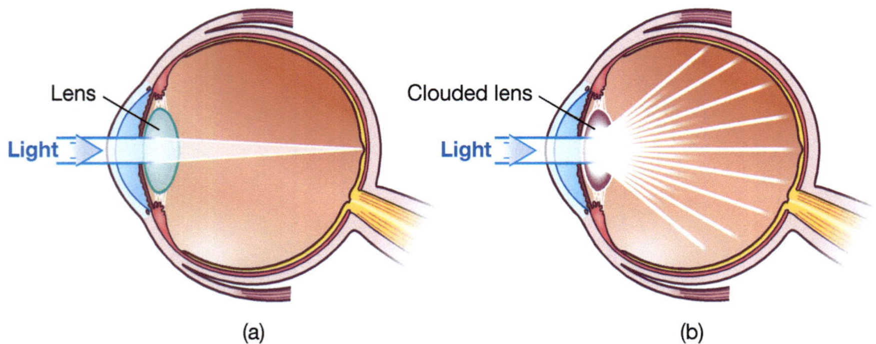

FIGURE 4.2 (a) Normal lens and (b) lens affected by cataract

When hearing the term cataract, it can be thought of as a metaphor for something that blocks clear vision. In the eye, this condition involves the lens becoming cloudy, which impairs the person's ability to see clearly. Understanding this origin can help you better grasp why the term is used in the context of eye care.

Cataracts come in various types, each affecting the eye's lens differently. Understanding these types helps in diagnosing and managing the condition effectively. Table 4.1 provides a breakdown of the different types of cataracts.

Table 4.1 Types of cataracts

Type of cataract	Symptoms	Progression/management
Nuclear cataracts: These cataracts form in the centre (nucleus) of the lens. They are commonly associated with ageing.	Patients often experience gradual loss of vision and may notice that their vision becomes more yellow or brownish.	They tend to develop slowly and can eventually lead to significant vision impairment, if not treated.
Cortical cataracts: These cataracts affect the outer edge (cortex) of the lens. They usually start as small, wedge-shaped opacities at the periphery of the lens.	They can cause blurred or distorted vision, particularly in bright light, and may lead to glare and difficulty with night vision.	They often progress gradually and vision can be affected as the opacities move towards the centre of the lens.
Posterior subcapsular cataracts: These cataracts form at the back of the lens, just under the lens capsule. They can develop more quickly than other types.	Patients may experience difficulty with reading and night vision and increased sensitivity to glare.	They can cause more noticeable vision problems even in the early stages compared to other types.
Congenital cataracts: These cataracts are present at birth or develop in early childhood. They can be hereditary or result from prenatal infections or other factors.	Vision problems may be apparent from a very young age and early diagnosis and treatment are crucial to prevent long-term vision impairment.	Early intervention is often necessary, including surgery to remove the cataract and corrective measures such as glasses or contact lenses.
Secondary cataracts: These cataracts develop as a result of other medical conditions or as a complication of eye surgery. They can occur after surgery for conditions such as glaucoma or after trauma.	Vision problems are similar to other cataracts, depending on their location and severity.	Often treated with additional surgery, including procedures such as yttrium aluminium garnet (YAG) laser capsulotomy to clear the clouded capsule. YAG laser, a type of laser commonly used in ophthalmology for various eye treatments.
Traumatic cataracts: Result from an injury to the eye. The trauma can cause the lens to become cloudy or opacified.	It can vary depending on the severity of the trauma, but generally includes vision impairment.	Treatment may involve surgery to remove the cataract and address any other damage caused by the injury.
Radiation cataracts: Develop after exposure to radiation, such as during radiation therapy for cancer.	Vision problems are similar to other cataract types, with the potential for rapid progression following radiation exposure.	Regular eye examinations are crucial for those who have undergone radiation therapy, with treatment focusing on cataract removal if necessary.

Source: Adapted from National Eye Institute (2023); Needham (2019).

Cataracts are categorised based on their location, causes and progression. Understanding the type of cataract is essential for determining the appropriate treatment approach. While nuclear and cortical cataracts are primarily age-related, other types, such as congenital, traumatic and secondary cataracts, may require specialised management. Identifying the type helps in planning effective interventions to improve vision and quality of life for patients.

PATHOPHYSIOLOGICAL CHANGES ASSOCIATED WITH CATARACT

A cataract is a congenital or degenerative opacity of the lens. It develops due to various pathophysiological changes in the lens of the eye, and they can form in one or both eyes (American Academy of Ophthalmology 2021). These changes are primarily related to the ageing process, but they can also be influenced by genetic factors, environmental exposures, systemic diseases and certain medications (see Table 4.2). An awareness of these changes provides insight into the mechanisms behind cataract formation and progression.

Table 4.2 Risk factors associated with cataract

Risk factor	Discussion
Age	Age is the most significant risk factor for cataracts. The prevalence of cataracts increases dramatically with age. Most individuals over the age of 60 years will experience some degree of lens clouding, with the risk continuing to rise as they grow older.
Genetics	Genetic predisposition (hereditary influence) plays a role in the development of cataracts. Individuals with a family history of cataracts are at higher risk. Certain genetic disorders, such as Down syndrome, are also associated with an increased incidence of cataracts.
Ultraviolet (UV) radiation	Prolonged exposure to UV radiation from the sun can increase the risk of cataracts. UV rays cause oxidative stress and damage to the lens proteins, leading to their aggregation and clouding over time.
Smoking	Tobacco use significantly increases the risk of cataract formation. Smokers are at a higher risk of developing nuclear cataracts, which affect the centre of the lens. The toxins in cigarette smoke cause oxidative damage to the lens.
Alcohol consumption	Chronic alcohol consumption has been linked to an elevated risk of cataracts. Alcohol can deplete antioxidants in the body, contributing to oxidative stress and lens damage.
Medical conditions	Diabetes: People with diabetes are at a higher risk of developing cataracts. High blood glucose levels can lead to the accumulation of sorbitol in the lens, causing swelling and clouding. Hypertension: High blood pressure has also been associated with an increased risk of cataracts. Obesity: Excessive body weight can increase the risk due to associated metabolic and vascular complications.
Medications	Long-term use of corticosteroid medications can increase the risk of posterior subcapsular cataracts. These medications are often prescribed for chronic inflammatory conditions. Other drugs: Certain medications, such as phenothiazine-related antipsychotics and statins, have also been linked to an increased risk of cataract development.

Risk factor	Discussion
Eye disease	Secondary cataract may develop as a complication of another eye disease, including chronic anterior uveitis, acute congestive angle-closure glaucoma, high myopia (a severe form of near-sightedness) and some hereditary fundus dystrophies (inherited disorders affecting the retina, leading to progressive vision loss).
Eye injuries	Trauma or physical injury to the eye can lead to traumatic cataracts. These cataracts can form immediately after the injury or develop years later. Penetrating eye injuries, blunt trauma and exposure to certain chemicals are common causes.
Radiation exposure	Exposure to ionising radiation, such as from X-rays or cancer treatments, can increase the risk of cataracts. This type of radiation causes damage to the lens cells, leading to opacity.
Nutritional deficiencies	A diet lacking in antioxidants, vitamins (especially vitamins C and E) and minerals can increase the risk of cataracts. Antioxidants help neutralise free radicals that can damage the lens proteins.
Gender and ethnicity	Gender: Women are at a slightly higher risk of developing cataracts compared to men, possibly due to hormonal differences and longer life expectancy. Ethnicity: Certain ethnic groups have a higher prevalence of cataracts and may develop them earlier than Caucasians.
Other environmental factors	Pollution: Exposure to environmental pollutants, including heavy metals and industrial chemicals, can increase the risk of cataract formation. Lifestyle factors: Prolonged exposure to heat and frequent use of certain electronic devices without proper eye protection might contribute to an increased risk.

Source: Adapted from British Medical Journal (2018); Galloway et al. (2022).

PROTEIN AGGREGATION AND CRYSTALLIN CHANGES

The lens is made up of water and proteins, primarily crystallins, which are crucial for maintaining the transparency and refractive properties of the lens. With age or due to metabolic disruptions (e.g. diabetes), crystallins can denature and aggregate, forming protein clumps. These aggregates scatter light, leading to the cloudiness characteristic of cataracts. Post-translational modifications (chemical changes to proteins after they are made) such as glycation, oxidation and deamidation can alter crystallin structure and function, promoting aggregation.

OXIDATIVE STRESS AND FREE RADICAL DAMAGE

The lens is continuously exposed to oxidative stress from ultraviolet (UV) light and metabolic processes, leading to ongoing damage from both UV exposure and bodily functions. Over time, the lens loses some of its natural defences, such as antioxidants, which makes it more vulnerable as ageing occurs. Harmful molecules called reactive oxygen species can damage parts of cells, for example, fats, proteins and DNA, leading to the lens becoming cloudy.

WATER AND ION IMBALANCE

In conditions such as diabetes, high glucose levels in the eye's fluid are turned into sorbitol by a specific enzyme. Sorbitol then makes water enter the lens, causing it to swell and become cloudy. If the mechanisms that control ion movement in the lens (Na^+/K^+ ATPase pump) do not work properly, this disrupts the lens's balance and can lead to cataracts.

LENS FIBRE CELL CHANGES

Cell differentiation occurs when lens cells change as they mature, losing organelles and other components to maintain transparency. However, in cataracts, this process is disrupted, leading to the accumulation of damaged proteins and cloudiness in the lens. Ageing and other issues can dysregulate this process. Damage from stress and metabolic problems (fibre cell integrity) affects the lens cells, making it less clear.

GENETIC AND MOLECULAR FACTORS

Changes in genes that produce lens proteins or control lens functions (genetic mutations) can increase the risk of developing cataracts. Normally, specific enzymes break down proteins in a controlled way. If these enzymes are not performing effectively, it can lead to improper breakdown of proteins. This can cause proteins to clump together in the lens of the eye, which can contribute to cataracts.

ENVIRONMENTAL AND LIFESTYLE FACTORS

Prolonged exposure to UV radiation from sunlight increases the risk of cataract formation due to oxidative damage. Both smoking and excessive alcohol consumption have been linked to increased oxidative stress and higher cataract risk.

SYSTEMIC DISEASES AND MEDICATIONS

Diabetes is a significant risk factor due to hyperglycaemia-induced changes in lens metabolism. Long-term use of corticosteroids can lead to posterior subcapsular cataracts due to changes in lens protein and cell metabolism.

The three most common types of cataracts are nuclear, cortical and posterior subcapsular. Less common are anterior subcapsular, anterior polar and posterior polar cataracts (American Academy of Ophthalmology 2021). Cataracts form due to a mix of protein clumping, oxidative stress, water imbalance, genetic factors and lifestyle influences. Understanding these changes helps in creating prevention and treatment strategies to manage cataracts and keep the lens clear.

EPIDEMIOLOGY

Cataracts are the leading cause of blindness worldwide (World Health Organization 2023). Hashemi, Pakzad, and Yekta (2020) report that around 36 million people worldwide are blind and in over 12 million of them, this is due to cataracts.

Data from multiple studies have been combined to find out how common age-related cataracts are worldwide and in different regions. They adjusted for age differences in the populations studied and found that 17.2% of people have cataracts. This adjustment allows for a fair comparison across regions with different age distributions. The study by Hashemi, Pakzad, and Yekta (2020) provided these estimates:

- 20–39 years was 3.01%

- 40–59 years was 16.97%

- Over 60 years was 54.38%

These values were, respectively:

- 2.18, 7.26 and 24.78% for cortical cataract

- 1.12, 5.77 and 31.19% for nuclear cataract

- 0.52, 1.91 and 7.29% for posterior subcapsular cataract

Cataract surgery is the most common elective surgical procedure in the UK, as reported by the Royal College of Ophthalmologists in 2018. The surgical procedure to remove cataracts involves replacing the cloudy lens with an artificial intraocular lens (IOL), significantly improving vision and quality of life for patients.

Cataract surgery is especially prevalent among the elderly population. As the UK's population ages, the demand for this surgery has been steadily increasing. It is estimated that around 400 000 cataract operations are performed each year in the UK, making it not only the most common but also one of the most successful surgical procedures (Stanford 2023). According to data from the Royal College of Ophthalmologists, the incidence of cataracts requiring surgery is highest among those in their 70s and 80s. Women tend to undergo cataract surgery more often than men, a trend that is attributed to women generally having a longer life expectancy and consequently, a higher likelihood of developing cataracts.

RISK FACTORS

Cataracts develop due to various factors that contribute to the clouding of the eye's natural lens. Understanding these risk factors can help prevent or delay the onset of cataracts and improve eye health outcomes. The risk factors are highlighted in Table 4.2.

Understanding the risk factors associated with cataracts is essential for preventing the condition, promoting early detection and intervention, improving patient care, guiding public health strategies, reducing healthcare costs and improving overall quality of life. Through awareness and targeted actions, both individuals and healthcare providers can work together to manage and mitigate the impact of cataracts on society.

CLINICAL PRESENTATION

Cataracts develop gradually, and their clinical presentation varies depending on the type and severity of the lens opacity. Symptoms can range from subtle vision changes to significant visual impairment. Understanding these symptoms is crucial for early diagnosis and appropriate management.

BLURRED VISION

The most common and earliest symptom of cataracts is progressively blurred or cloudy vision. This occurs because the cataract scatters and blocks light as it passes through the lens, preventing a clear image from reaching the retina. Patients often describe their vision as looking through a foggy or frosted window.

DIFFICULTY WITH NIGHT VISION

Cataracts can cause significant difficulty seeing in low-light conditions or at night (Needham 2019). This poor vision in low light is particularly noticeable when driving at night, where patients may experience halos or glare around headlights and streetlights. This symptom is often one of the first noticeable changes for individuals with early cataracts.

SENSITIVITY TO LIGHT AND GLARE

Increased sensitivity to light, known as photophobia, is a common complaint. Bright lights can cause discomfort and glare, making it challenging to see clearly in well-lit environments. This sensitivity can be particularly troublesome when transitioning from dark to bright areas.

HALOS AROUND LIGHTS

Many individuals with cataracts report seeing halos around lights (visual disturbances), especially at night. These halos can appear as rings of light surrounding bright objects and are caused by the scattering of light within the cloudy lens (National Institute for Health and Care Excellence [NICE] 2017).

FADING OR YELLOWING OF COLOURS

Cataracts can affect colour perception, causing colours to appear faded or yellow (colour perception changes), (Galloway et al. 2022). This occurs because the lens, which helps filter light, becomes discoloured with age, altering how colours are perceived. Patients may have difficulty distinguishing between shades of the same colour or notice a general dullness in their visual environment.

DOUBLE VISION IN ONE EYE

Monocular diplopia, or double vision in one eye, can occur due to cataracts. This type of double vision is different from binocular diplopia, which occurs when both eyes are misaligned. Monocular diplopia persists even when the other eye is covered. This symptom is caused by irregularities in the lens surface due to cataracts (Sanderson 2019).

FREQUENT PRESCRIPTION CHANGES

As the cataract progresses, it can alter the refractive power of the lens, leading to rapid shifts in vision clarity. Frequent prescription changes can be a sign of cataract progression, as the condition causes changes in the lens that affect its refractive properties. These refractive stability issues lead to fluctuating vision, necessitating regular updates to corrective lenses

(Sanderson 2019). Regular eye examinations and monitoring are essential to manage these changes effectively. Ultimately, cataract surgery can provide a long-term solution, restoring clear and stable vision.

DIFFICULTY READING

Near-vision problems can occur. Cataracts can make it challenging to read small print or perform tasks that require fine visual acuity. This is particularly problematic for tasks such as reading, sewing or working on a computer. Patients may find themselves needing brighter light or magnifying lenses to read comfortably.

As cataracts progress, they can significantly impact daily activities such as driving, reading, recognising faces and performing tasks that require fine visual detail. This can lead to a loss of independence and affect the overall quality of life.

Recognising the clinical presentation of cataracts is crucial for early diagnosis and timely intervention. Blurred vision, difficulty with night vision, sensitivity to light and changes in colour perception are common symptoms that should prompt a thorough eye examination. Early detection and management can significantly improve visual outcomes and quality of life for individuals with cataracts.

CLINICAL INVESTIGATIONS AND DIAGNOSIS

Diagnosis is usually based on self-reported symptoms and a series of tests performed by an optometrist, normally based in the community. A systematic and thorough approach to diagnosis is advocated, which usually entails a patient history and a range of comprehensive eye examinations. It is imperative that the person offering care and support to people with cataracts adheres to local policies and procedures concerning infection prevention and control, consent and the use of chaperones.

PATIENT HISTORY

History taking is a key component of the diagnostic process for cataracts, establishing if one or both eyes are affected. It provides essential information about the patient's symptoms, medical background, lifestyle and risk factors that contribute to the development and progression of cataracts. The following aspects are relevant to history taking and cataracts.

Chief Complaint   This begins with understanding the patient's symptoms:
Blurry vision: When did the patient first notice a decrease in vision clarity?
Glare and light sensitivity: Is the patient experiencing sensitivity to light or glare, particularly when driving at night?
Colour perception changes: Has the patient noticed a fading or yellowing of colours?
Double vision: Is there a presence of double vision in one eye (monocular diplopia)?

Onset and Duration   The timing and progression of symptoms are determined:
Acute versus chronic: Did the symptoms come on suddenly or gradually?
Progressive nature: How have the symptoms evolved over time? Are they worsening steadily?

Impact on Daily Activities   Ascertain functional impairment:
Reading difficulties: Is reading becoming more challenging? Does the patient need brighter light or magnification?

Driving issues: Are there specific problems with night driving or seeing street signs?
Work and hobbies: Are vision problems interfering with work, hobbies or other daily activities?

Previous Eye Health Discuss past ocular history, the patient is asked about:
Previous eye conditions: Has the patient been diagnosed with other eye conditions such as glaucoma, macular degeneration or diabetic retinopathy?
Eye surgery or injuries: Any history of eye surgery (including laser-assisted in situ keratomileusis [LASIK] or photorefractive keratectomy [PRK]) or significant eye injuries?
Use of corrective lenses: How long has the patient been using glasses or contact lenses? Any recent changes in prescription?

Systemic Health and Medications Here the patient's general health status is assessed:
Chronic diseases: Does the patient have systemic conditions, for example, diabetes, hypertension or autoimmune diseases that can affect eye health?
Medications: A detailed list of current medications, especially corticosteroids, which can accelerate cataract formation.
Smoking and alcohol use: These habits are significant risk factors for cataracts.

Family History Genetic predisposition:
Family history of cataracts: Are there any family members with a history of cataracts or other hereditary eye conditions?
Other eye diseases: Any genetic conditions known to affect eye health?

Occupational and Lifestyle Factors An overview of environmental and lifestyle influences is discussed:
Exposure to UV radiation: Does the patient spend significant time outdoors or in environments with high UV exposure without adequate eye protection?
Occupational hazards: Any exposure to radiation, chemicals or other hazards that could affect eye health?
Diet and nutrition: Inquiry about diet, particularly the intake of nutrients such as vitamins A, C and E, which are important for eye health.

Review of Systems A comprehensive health overview is undertaken:
Systemic symptoms: The patient is asked about symptoms in other body systems that can provide clues about underlying health conditions that may affect the eyes.
Overall well-being: General health and well-being can impact eye health and the patient's ability to undergo and recover from potential cataract surgery.

Patient Concerns and Expectations Adopt a patient-centred approach. What are the patient's main concerns regarding their vision and eye health? Discuss what the patient hopes to achieve with treatment, particularly if cataract surgery is being considered.

History taking is an initial step in diagnosing cataracts, offering critical insight into the patient's symptoms, medical background and lifestyle factors. A thorough history helps guide the clinical examination, identify potential risk factors and develop a personalised management plan. Effective history taking ensures a comprehensive understanding of the patient's condition, facilitating early diagnosis and appropriate intervention to preserve vision and quality of life.

EXAMINATION AND INVESTIGATIONS

Diagnosing cataracts involves a series of clinical investigations; these investigations help to confirm the presence of cataracts, determine their severity and plan appropriate treatment. The patient is usually referred to an optometrist who performs an eye examination and measures visual acuity to make a confirmation of the diagnosis and to exclude other causes of visual impairment. Co-existing eye conditions, for example, glaucoma, age-related macular degeneration, diabetic retinopathy and amblyopia, may also be present in those who require cataract surgery.

Guidance concerning investigations and examination is available through NICE (2017) and other national level organisations. Table 4.3 provides an overview of a range of investigations and examinations to make a diagnosis of cataract; the choice of investigation is based on patient need and local protocol.

Table 4.3 Examinations and investigations

Examination	Discussion
Comprehensive eye examination	This is the first step in diagnosing cataracts and typically includes the following components: Visual acuity test: Measures how well a patient can see at various distances. Reduced visual acuity can indicate the presence of cataracts. Refraction test: This test determines the exact prescription needed for corrective lenses. By using a phoropter or autorefractor, how light waves are bent as they pass through the cornea and lens are measured. Frequent changes in prescription can be a sign of cataract development.
Slit-lamp examination	Slit-lamp biomicroscopy: A slit-lamp examination provides a magnified, three-dimensional view of the structures at the front of the eye, including the cornea, iris, lens and anterior chamber. By shining a thin beam of light into the eye, the ophthalmologist can closely examine the lens for any signs of opacities or cloudiness indicative of cataracts.
Retinal examination	Dilated eye examination: In this procedure, the ophthalmologist uses eye drops to dilate (widen) the pupils. This allows for a better view of the retina at the back of the eye using an ophthalmoscope or a slit lamp with special lenses. The dilated eye examination helps in assessing the overall health of the retina and identifying any other conditions that might be contributing to vision problems.
Contrast sensitivity test	Evaluating visual function: Contrast sensitivity testing measures the ability to distinguish between different shades of light and dark. This is particularly useful in detecting cataracts that may not significantly affect visual acuity but still impair the quality of vision by reducing contrast sensitivity.

(Continued)

Table 4.3 (*Continued*)

Examination	Discussion
Glare testing	Assessing light sensitivity:
	Glare testing evaluates how well the eyes function under bright light conditions. Since cataracts can cause significant glare and light sensitivity, this test helps to quantify the impact on vision.
Tonometry	Measuring intraocular pressure:
	Although not directly related to cataracts, tonometry measures the pressure inside the eye. This is important because high intraocular pressure can indicate glaucoma, which may coexist with cataracts and require simultaneous management.
Optical coherence tomography (OCT)	Detailed retinal imaging:
	OCT provides high-resolution, cross-sectional images of the retina. This imaging test helps in detecting any macular diseases or retinal detachment, which can affect the treatment plan for cataracts.
A-scan ultrasound biometry	Measuring eye structures:
	An A-scan ultrasound measures the length of the eye and the curvature of the cornea. These measurements are crucial for calculating the power of the intraocular lens to be implanted during cataract surgery.
Specular microscopy	Corneal endothelial cell analysis:
	This test assesses the endothelial cells on the back surface of the cornea. It is important for patients with coexisting corneal conditions, as it helps determine the health of the cornea before cataract surgery.

Source: Adapted from NICE (2017), Needham (2019), Sanderson (2019) and Galloway et al. (2022).

A thorough clinical investigation is essential for the accurate diagnosis of cataracts. This process includes a comprehensive eye examination, slit-lamp examination, retinal assessment and various specialised tests. Early and precise diagnosis allows for timely and effective treatment, helping to preserve vision and improve the quality of life for patients with cataracts.

MANAGEMENT

Cataract management usually involves a multidisciplinary team that includes ophthalmologists, optometrists, nurses and technicians with the patient at the centre of all that is done. In those adults with early age-related cataracts, a non-surgical management approach may include prescription of spectacles (refractive correction). The provision of brighter lighting for tasks such as reading can reduce the impact of cataracts on daily activities. Alternatively, adults with age-related cataracts may be referred for surgery by an optometrist or a general practitioner. The clinical threshold used to access cataract surgery varies (NICE 2017).

The decision to undergo cataract surgery must be based on a discussion with the patient (and if appropriate, their family or carers). The discussion includes:

- How cataract affects the person's vision and their quality of life.

- Whether one or both eyes are affected.

- What the surgery involves, including the risks and benefits. Care is required when returning home.

- Whether they want to have surgery.

- How their quality of life may be affected if they choose not to have surgery.

The Royal College of Ophthalmologists and Royal National Institute of Blind People (2022) have produced literature that can help people be part of the decision-making process regarding treatment options.

SURGICAL MANAGEMENT

Surgery is the primary treatment for cataracts, especially when they cause significant visual impairment or affect daily living. The UK has provided established protocols for cataract surgery.

CATARACT SURGERY PROCEDURE

Preoperative assessment: This includes measuring eye parameters (e.g. axial length, corneal curvature) to select the appropriate IOL. The aim of cataract surgery is to provide patients with the best possible vision. Patients can expect to gain functional near and far vision (Stanford 2023).

Surgical technique: Most commonly performed using phacoemulsification, where the cloudy lens is broken up using ultrasound and then removed through a small incision. A new artificial lens (IOL) is then implanted. See Figure 4.3.

Local anaesthesia: Typically performed under local anaesthesia with sedation, the patient is awake but the eye is numb.

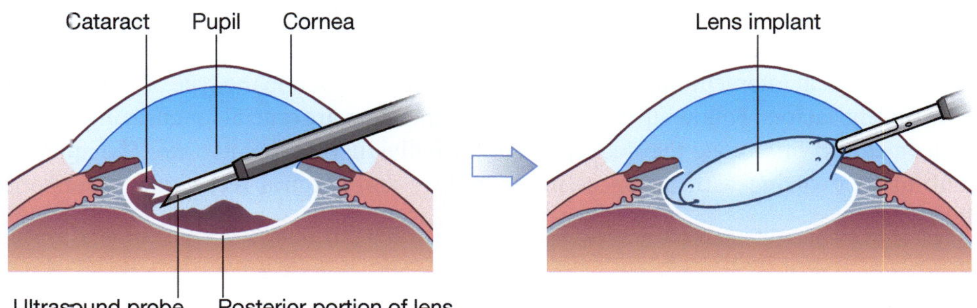

FIGURE 4.3   Phacoemulsification

TYPES OF INTRA-OPTICAL LENSES

- Monofocal intra-optical lenses: Provide clear vision at one distance (usually distance vision). Patients may still need glasses for reading or close work.

- Multifocal intra-optical lenses: Allow for vision at multiple distances (near, intermediate and far), reducing the need for glasses.

- Accommodating intra-optical lenses: Designed to mimic the eye's natural focusing ability and provide a range of vision.

POSTOPERATIVE CARE

Patients may expect their eye to be covered with a plastic shield known as a cartella, especially if there are residual effects from the local anaesthesia (NICE 2017). The cartella protects the eye because the patient may not feel any debris, such as dust, that could enter the eye. The decision to use a cartella postoperatively often depends on surgeon preference. Patients discharged with a cartella can remove and discard it the following morning or as instructed in their postoperative care information.

In the initial postoperative phase, patients may experience a gritty sensation in the eye and sensitivity to bright light. The eyelids may be bruised and the conjunctiva (the white part of the eye) might appear red. Postoperative eye cleansing is generally not necessary, unless advised otherwise in the postoperative instructions. If there is slight 'crustiness' the morning after surgery, some patients may be provided with sterile, non-linting swabs, normal saline, a sterile gallipot and a pack of sterile swabs in their discharge pack. Alternatively, cooled boiled water may be recommended instead of normal saline for cleaning the eye (Stanford 2023).

RECOVERY AND FOLLOW-UP

Patients are usually discharged on the same day as surgery. Postoperative care includes using prescribed eye drops to prevent infection and inflammation. Follow-up visits are scheduled to monitor the healing process and ensure that the eye is recovering as expected.

Potential complications such as infection, inflammation or posterior capsule opacification (PCO) are managed promptly. PCO, also known as secondary cataract, can be treated with a procedure called YAG laser capsulotomy.

The management of cataracts involves a comprehensive approach from diagnosis to postoperative care, guided by NICE guidelines and best practices. The primary treatment for cataracts is surgical intervention, with careful consideration given to the type of IOL used and patient-specific factors. Follow-up care and patient education are crucial for ensuring successful outcomes and improving the quality of life for individuals with cataracts. The approach is continually evolving with advances in technology and surgical techniques to enhance patient outcomes.

HEALTH TEACHING

Health teaching for people with cataracts involves providing patients with information about the condition, treatment options, postoperative care, lifestyle adjustments, infection prevention and control and preventive measures. Effective education helps patients make informed decisions, manage their condition better and improve their overall quality of life. Any information or advice provided by those who offer care and support must be tailored to meet the needs of the individual patient. Table 4.4 outlines the health teaching needs of people with cataracts.

Health teaching for people with cataracts is comprehensive and involves the provision of information about the condition, its management and preventive measures. Through information giving and advice provision, patients can better understand their condition, make informed decisions about their care and adopt healthy lifestyle changes to support their eye health and overall well-being. Infection prevention and control are critical components of postoperative care to ensure successful outcomes and minimise complications.

Table 4.4 Health teaching needs of people with cataracts

Health education need	Discussion
Understanding cataracts	Offer the person definitions and symptoms associated with cataract.
	What is a cataract? A cataract is the clouding of the eye's natural lens, leading to a decrease in vision.
	Common symptoms: Blurry vision, difficulty with glare (especially at night), faded colours and frequent changes in eyeglass prescription.
	Causes and risk factors:
	Ageing: The most common cause.
	Other risk factors: Diabetes, prolonged exposure to sunlight, smoking, obesity, high blood pressure, previous eye injury or inflammation and certain medications (e.g. steroids).
Treatment options	Non-surgical management:
	Eyeglasses/contact lenses: May help in the early stages.
	Improved lighting: Using brighter lights at home or work.
	Magnifying lenses: For reading and other close-up tasks.
	Surgical management:
	When is surgery needed? If cataracts significantly impair vision and affect daily activities.
	Types of surgery: The most common is phacoemulsification with intraocular lens implantation.
	Benefits and risks: Offer information about the high success rate and potential risks including infection, bleeding and retinal detachment.
Preoperative education	Preparation for surgery:
	Medications: Instructions on which medications to continue or discontinue before surgery.
	Fasting: Guidelines on fasting before the surgery (refer to local policy and procedure).
	Transportation: Arrange for someone to accompany the patient home after the procedure.

(Continued)

Table 4.4 (*Continued*)

Health education need	Discussion
Postoperative care	Immediate post-surgery:
	Eye protection: Use of a plastic shield (cartella) to protect the eye, typically until the following morning.
	Eye drops: Instructions on using prescribed antibiotic and anti-inflammatory eye drops to prevent infection and reduce inflammation.
	Normal symptoms: Mild discomfort, grittiness, sensitivity to light, bruising of the eyelids and redness of the conjunctiva.
Infection prevention and control	Importance:
	Preventing infection is crucial for optimal healing and to avoid complications after cataract surgery.
	Hand hygiene:
	Before touching the eye: Always wash hands thoroughly with soap and water before touching the eye or administering eye drops.
	Eye drop administration:
	Sterile technique: Ensure that the tip of the eye drop bottle does not touch the eye or any other surface to maintain sterility.
	Proper usage: Follow the prescribed regimen strictly to prevent infection and promote healing.
	Avoid contaminants:
	Avoid dust and smoke: Keep the environment clean and avoid exposure to dust, smoke and other potential contaminants.
	Avoid swimming: Refrain from swimming in pools, hot tubs or natural bodies of water for at least two weeks post-surgery to reduce the risk of infection.
	Eye protection:
	Use of eye shield: Continue using the protective eye shield at night for the first week to avoid accidental rubbing or injury during sleep.
	Monitor for signs of infection:
	Symptoms to watch for: Increased redness, swelling, pain, discharge or a significant decrease in vision should be reported to the ophthalmologist immediately.
Activity restrictions	Avoid rubbing the eye:
	Prevents injury and reduces the risk of introducing bacteria.
	Limitations:
	Heavy lifting and strenuous activities: Avoid for a specified period.
	Showering/bathing: Take care to avoid water splashing into the eye.

Health education need	Discussion
Follow-up visits	Importance:
	Regular follow-ups to monitor healing and ensure no complications arise.
	Timely reporting: Report any concerns or unusual symptoms to the ophthalmologist promptly.
Lifestyle adjustments and preventive measures	Healthy diet:
	Antioxidants: Emphasise the importance of a diet rich in antioxidants (fruits and vegetables) to support eye health.
	Hydration: Staying well-hydrated.
	UV protection:
	Sunglasses: Wear sunglasses that block 100% of UV rays when outdoors.
	Regular eye examinations:
	Routine check-ups: Encourage regular eye examinations to monitor eye health, especially for individuals over 60 years or with risk factors.
Managing systemic conditions	Diabetes and hypertension: Controlling chronic conditions such as diabetes and high blood pressure to reduce the risk of developing cataracts.
	Smoking cessation:
	Quitting smoking: Advise patients to stop smoking, as it is a significant risk factor for cataracts.

Source: Galloway et al. (2022), Sanderson (2019), Needham (2019) and NICE (2017).

CONCLUSION

Cataracts represent a significant health concern, particularly among the ageing population, impacting visual acuity and quality of life. The comprehensive management of cataracts involves early detection through regular eye examinations, understanding the risk factors and timely intervention. Health education plays a pivotal role in empowering patients with knowledge about cataract formation, progression and the importance of lifestyle adjustments to delay onset and manage symptoms.

The primary treatment for cataracts is surgical, with phacoemulsification and IOL implantation being the most common and effective procedures. Advances in surgical techniques and IOL technology have significantly improved outcomes, allowing patients to regain clear vision and enhance their daily living.

Postoperative care, including the use of protective eye shields, administration of prescribed eye drops and adherence to activity restrictions, is crucial for successful recovery and infection prevention. Regular follow-up appointments ensure that any complications are promptly addressed and the patient's vision is monitored for stability and improvement.

Preventive measures, such as UV protection, a diet rich in antioxidants and managing systemic conditions such as diabetes, contribute to reducing the risk of cataract formation. Smoking cessation and minimising exposure to harmful environmental factors are also vital components of preventive health strategies.

A multifaceted approach that includes patient education, timely surgical intervention, diligent postoperative care and preventive lifestyle choices is essential in the effective management of cataracts. Through collaborative efforts between healthcare providers and patients, the burden of cataracts can be significantly reduced, allowing individuals to maintain optimal vision and independence as they age.

GLOSSARY OF TERMS

Accommodating intraocular lenses: A type of intraocular lens designed to mimic the eye's natural focusing ability, providing a range of vision from near to far.

Antioxidants: Substances that can prevent or slow damage to cells caused by free radicals. Common antioxidants include vitamins C and E, which are beneficial for eye health.

Axial length: The distance from the front to the back of the eye, important for calculating the power of the intraocular lens needed in cataract surgery.

Capsule: The membrane that surrounds the natural lens of the eye. In cataract surgery, the front part of the capsule is removed, but the back part remains to support the intraocular lens.

Cataract: The clouding of the eye's natural lens, which leads to a decrease in vision.

Conjunctiva: The clear, thin membrane that covers the white part of the eye and the inside of the eyelids.

Diplopia: Double vision, which can occur due to cataracts causing light to scatter inside the eye.

Glare: Difficulty seeing in the presence of bright light, a common symptom of cataracts.

Intraocular lens: An artificial lens implanted in the eye to replace the natural lens removed during cataract surgery.

Laser: A device that generates a concentrated beam of light, used in procedures such as yttrium aluminium garnet (YAG) laser capsulotomy to treat secondary cataracts.

LASIK: A type of refractive surgery to correct vision problems by reshaping the cornea.

Lens: The transparent structure inside the eye that focuses light onto the retina. In cataract surgery, the natural lens is replaced with an artificial lens.

Monofocal intraocular lenses: Intraocular lenses that provide clear vision at one distance, usually distance vision, requiring glasses for near tasks.

Multifocal intraocular lenses: Intraocular lenses designed to provide clear vision at multiple distances, reducing the need for glasses.

Myopia: Near-sightedness, a condition where distant objects appear blurry.

Phacoemulsification: A modern cataract surgery technique using ultrasound to break up and remove the cloudy lens.

Posterior capsule opacification: A common complication after cataract surgery where the back of the lens capsule becomes cloudy, affecting vision.

Refractive correction: Adjusting vision problems using glasses or contact lenses.

Slit-lamp examination: A diagnostic procedure where a microscope with a bright light is used to examine the eye.

Steroids: Medications that reduce inflammation, sometimes used in eye treatments but can increase the risk of cataracts with prolonged use.

UV protection: Measures to protect the eyes from ultraviolet light, which can help prevent cataracts.

Visual acuity: The clarity or sharpness of vision, often measured by reading letters on a chart.

YAG: A crystal used in lasers for medical procedures, including ophthalmology.

YAG laser capsulotomy: A procedure using a YAG laser to create an opening in the cloudy posterior capsule of the lens to restore clear vision after cataract surgery.

MULTIPLE CHOICE QUESTIONS

1. What is a cataract?
    a) Inflammation of the eye
    b) Clouding of the eye's natural lens
    c) Infection in the cornea
    d) Increase in intraocular pressure

2. Which of the following is a common symptom of cataracts?
    a) Redness in the eyes
    b) Pain in the eyes
    c) Blurry vision
    d) Eye twitching

3. Which type of cataract surgery is most commonly performed?
    a) LASIK
    b) PRK
    c) Phacoemulsification
    d) Vitrectomy

4. What is an intraocular lens?
    a) A lens worn on the outside of the eye
    b) A lens implanted inside the eye to replace the natural lens
    c) A lens that corrects corneal defects
    d) A temporary lens used during surgery

5. Which risk factor is most commonly associated with the development of cataracts?
    a) Young age
    b) Frequent eye infections
    c) Ageing
    d) Low blood pressure

6. What should patients avoid doing immediately after cataract surgery?
    a) Watching TV
    b) Reading
    c) Heavy lifting and bending
    d) Taking showers

7. Which condition can increase the risk of developing cataracts?
   a) Hypotension
   b) Diabetes
   c) Astigmatism
   d) Myopia

8. A cloudy appearance in which part of the eye is a sign of cataracts?
   a) Cornea
   b) Retina
   c) Lens
   d) Iris

9. Which of the following is not typically used to manage cataracts?
   a) Eyeglasses
   b) Contact lenses
   c) Anti-inflammatory medication
   d) Surgery

10. UV protection is important in preventing cataracts because:
    a) UV light directly damages the retina
    b) UV light causes clouding of the cornea
    c) UV light can accelerate the clouding of the lens
    d) UV light causes glaucoma

REFERENCES

American Academy of Ophthalmology (2021). *Cataract in the Adult Eye Preferred Practice Pattern*. San Francisco: American Academy of Ophthalmology.

British Medical Journal (2018). Cataracts. http://www.bestpractice.bmj.com.

Galloway, N.R., Amoaku, W.M., Galloway, P.H. et al. (2022). *Common Eye Diseases and Their Management*, 5e. London: Springer.

Hashemi, H., Pakzad, R., and Yekta, A. (2020). Global and regional prevalence of age-related cataract: a comprehensive systematic review and meta-analysis. *Eye* 34 (8): 1357–1370. doi: 10.1038/s41433-020-0806-3.

National Eye Institute (2023). Types of cataracts. https://www.nei.nih.gov/learn-about-eye-health/eye-conditions-and-diseases/cataracts/types-cataract (accessed July 2024).

National Institute for Health and Care Excellence (2017). Cataracts in adults: management. https://www.nice.org.uk/guidance/ng77/resources/cataracts-in-adults-management-pdf-1837639266757 (accessed July 2024).

Needham, Y. (2019). Ophthalmological disorders (Chapter 38). In: *Learning to Care* (ed. I. Peate). London: Elsevier.

Royal College of Ophthalmologists and Royal National Institute of Blind People (2022). Understanding cataracts. https://www.rcophth.ac.uk/wp-content/uploads/2023/03/Understanding-Cataracts-2022.pdf (accessed July 2024).

Sanderson, A. (2019). Nursing patients with disorders of the eye and sight impairment (Chapter 14). In: *Alexander's Nursing Practice*, 5e (ed. I. Peate), London: Elsevier.

Stanford, P. (2023). Cataracts: the essentials for patient care. *British Journal of Community Nursing* 28 (5): 230–236.

World Health Organization (2023). Blindness and vision impairment. https://www.who.int/news-room/fact-sheets/detail/blindness-and-visual-impairment (accessed July 2024).

Conjunctivitis CHAPTER 5

PINK EYE

Conjunctivitis, commonly known as 'pink eye', is an inflammation or infection of the conjunctiva, the transparent membrane that lines the eyelid and covers the white part of the eyeball. This is a contagious condition. There are several types of conjunctivitis, each with different causes and treatments (Galloway et al. 2022).

VIRAL CONJUNCTIVITIS

- **Cause:** Most commonly caused by adenoviruses, but other viruses such as herpes simplex virus can also be responsible.

- **Symptoms:** Watery discharge, redness, irritation and often starts in one eye before spreading to the other. It is highly contagious.

- **Treatment:** Usually this is self-limiting; antiviral medications may be prescribed for severe cases, especially if caused by herpes simplex. Cold compresses and artificial tears can help alleviate symptoms.

BACTERIAL CONJUNCTIVITIS

- **Cause:** Caused by bacteria such as *Staphylococcus aureus*, *Streptococcus pneumoniae* or *Haemophilus influenzae*. It can be caused by *Neisseria gonorrhoeae* or *Chlamydia trachomatis*.

- **Symptoms:** Thick, yellow-green discharge, redness, irritation and sometimes there may be eyelid swelling. Often affects both eyes.

- **Treatment:** Antibiotic eye drops or ointments are typically prescribed. Hygiene measures such as frequent hand washing can help prevent spreading infection.

ALLERGIC CONJUNCTIVITIS

- **Cause:** Triggered by allergens such as pollen, pet dander, dust mites or certain medications.

- **Symptoms:** Itchy eyes, redness, tearing and swelling of the eyelids. Often associated with other allergic symptoms such as sneezing and nasal congestion.

- **Treatment:** Avoiding allergens, using antihistamine or anti-inflammatory eye drops and sometimes oral antihistamines. Cold compress can also provide relief.

CHEMICAL CONJUNCTIVITIS

- **Cause:** Exposure to irritants such as smoke, chlorine in swimming pools, air pollutants or chemical fumes.

- **Symptoms:** Redness, watering, irritation and pain. Symptoms occur shortly after exposure to the irritant.

- **Treatment:** Immediate and thorough rinsing of the eyes with water or saline solution. Avoidance of the irritant is essential. Severe cases may require medical attention and the use of anti-inflammatory medications.

GIANT PAPILLARY CONJUNCTIVITIS

- **Cause:** Often associated with contact lens wear, especially if lenses are not cleaned properly or worn for extended periods. Can also be caused by the presence of a foreign body in the eye.

- **Symptoms:** Itching, redness, a mucous discharge and a feeling of something in the eye. The inner surface of the eyelid may develop large, raised bumps.

- **Treatment:** Discontinuing contact lens use, ensuring proper lens hygiene and using prescribed anti-inflammatory eye drops. Switching to daily disposable lenses may also help.

NEONATAL CONJUNCTIVITIS

- **Cause:** Newborns can acquire this type of conjunctivitis during birth if the mother has a sexually transmitted infection such as gonorrhoea or chlamydia.

- **Symptoms:** Redness, swelling of the eyelids and discharge, which can be severe.

- **Treatment:** Prompt medical treatment with appropriate antibiotics is crucial to prevent complications. Prophylactic eye drops are often given to newborns at birth to prevent this condition.

NON-INFECTIOUS CONJUNCTIVITIS

- **Cause:** Can result from mechanical irritation (e.g. a foreign body in the eye), contact lens wear or other non-infectious factors.

- **Symptoms:** Redness, irritation and tearing, without the typical signs of infection such as discharge.

- **Treatment:** Removing the irritant, improving contact lens hygiene and using lubricating eye drops. Anti-inflammatory drops may be prescribed in some cases.

PATHOPHYSIOLOGICAL CHANGES ASSOCIATED WITH CONJUNCTIVITIS

Conjunctivitis is an inflammation of the conjunctiva, the thin, transparent membrane covering the white part of the eye and the inner surface of the eyelids (see Figure 5.1). It is extremely prevalent in the general population; those who offer care and support to people in primary care settings often play a crucial role in diagnosing and managing this condition. Given the conjunctiva's constant exposure to environmental elements during waking hours, it is especially vulnerable to inflammation. This section will explore the pathophysiological changes that occur in conjunctivitis and the various causes and mechanisms behind them.

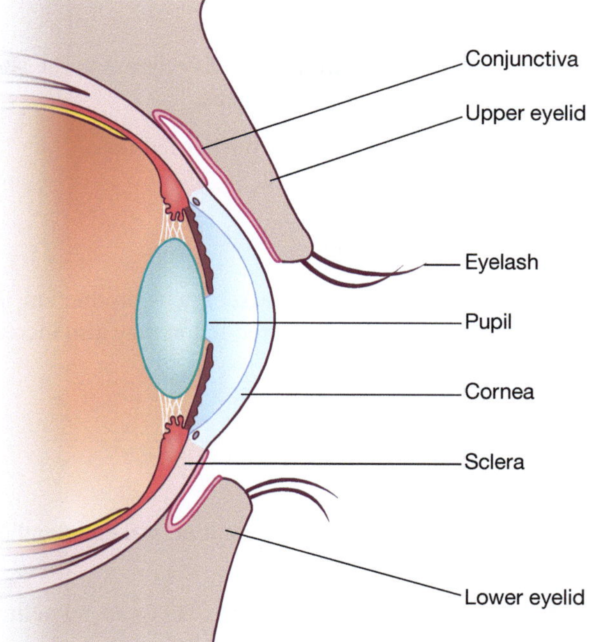

FIGURE 5.1   The eye and associated structures (the conjunctiva)

CONJUNCTIVAL ANATOMY AND FUNCTION

The conjunctiva serves several key functions:

- Protection: Acts as a barrier against pathogens and foreign bodies.

- Lubrication: Produces mucus and tears to keep the eye moist.

- Immune defence: Contains immune cells that respond to infections.

Given these functions, the conjunctiva is well-equipped to deal with environmental insults but can still become inflamed under certain conditions.

The pathophysiological changes in conjunctivitis vary depending on the underlying cause but generally include (Azari and Arabi 2020; Galloway et al. 2022):

VASODILATION AND INCREASED BLOOD FLOW

- In response to infection or irritation, the blood vessels in the conjunctiva dilate to increase blood flow.

- This causes the characteristic redness (hyperaemia) of the eye (clinical manifestation).

INCREASED VASCULAR PERMEABILITY

- Inflammatory mediators increase the permeability of conjunctival blood vessels, allowing immune cells and proteins to move into the tissue.

- This results in swelling (chemosis) and sometimes there is discharge from the eye.

IMMUNE CELL INFILTRATION

- Neutrophils, lymphocytes and other immune cells migrate to the site of inflammation in order to combat pathogens or respond to allergens.

- This can cause a gritty sensation, along with further redness.

MUCOUS AND TEAR PRODUCTION

- Goblet cells located in the conjunctiva increase mucus production. This mechanism is in response to irritation or infection and tear production may also increase.

- This leads to watery or mucoid discharge.

CELLULAR DAMAGE AND REPAIR

- Pathogens, allergens or irritants can damage conjunctival epithelial cells, triggering repair mechanisms.

- Damaged cells are sloughed off and replaced. This can sometimes cause temporary discomfort.

TYPES OF CONJUNCTIVITIS AND SPECIFIC PATHOPHYSIOLOGICAL MECHANISMS

VIRAL CONJUNCTIVITIS

- Cause: Most commonly adenoviruses.

- Pathophysiology: Virus infects epithelial cells, leading to cell lysis and immune response activation. Inflammatory mediators such as cytokines and chemokines are released. These attract immune cells.

BACTERIAL CONJUNCTIVITIS

- Cause: Bacteria such as *Staphylococcus aureus*, *Streptococcus pneumoniae*.

- Pathophysiology: Bacteria adhere to the conjunctival epithelium. This triggers an immune response. Neutrophils are predominant, leading to purulent discharge.

ALLERGIC CONJUNCTIVITIS

- Cause: Allergens, for example, pollen, pet dander.

- Pathophysiology: Allergen exposure leads to an IgE-mediated hypersensitivity reaction. Mast cells degranulate, releasing histamine and other mediators.

CHEMICAL CONJUNCTIVITIS

- Cause: Irritants such as smoke, chlorine.

- Pathophysiology: Chemical irritants cause direct damage to conjunctival cells and stimulate an inflammatory response.

GIANT PAPILLARY CONJUNCTIVITIS

- Cause: This is often associated with contact lens wear.

- Pathophysiology: Mechanical irritation from contact lenses or foreign bodies leads to chronic inflammation and formation of large papillae.

NEONATAL CONJUNCTIVITIS

- Cause: Typically from maternal infections (e.g. gonorrhoea, chlamydia).

- Pathophysiology: Bacteria infect the conjunctiva during birth, leading to an intense inflammatory response.

NON-INFECTIOUS CONJUNCTIVITIS

- Cause: Mechanical irritation, contact lens wear.

- Pathophysiology: Physical irritation leads to a mild inflammatory response.

PROTECTIVE MECHANISMS AND SELF-LIMITING NATURE

Despite the conjunctiva's exposure to potential infections, it has robust protective mechanisms. Tears contain immunoglobulins (especially IgA) and lysozyme, which have antimicrobial properties. Tears also help wash away debris and pathogens. Mucus traps particles and microorganisms, facilitating their removal from the eye. The conjunctiva has resident immune cells that can quickly respond to infections.

These protective mechanisms often lead to the self-limiting nature of conjunctivitis, especially in viral and mild bacterial cases. The immune response clears the infection and the epithelial cells repair any damage, restoring normal function.

Conjunctivitis is usually acute; however, both infectious and allergic conditions can be chronic Additional conditions that cause chronic conjunctivitis include:

- Ectropion (a condition in which the eyelid, typically the lower one, turns outward away from the eye).

- Entropion (a condition where the eyelid, typically the lower one, turns inward towards the eye).

- Blepharitis (inflammation of the eyelids, usually involving the part of the eyelid where the eyelashes grow).

- Chronic dacryocystitis (a persistent inflammation or infection of the lacrimal sac, which is part of the tear drainage system of the eye).

Conjunctivitis is a common condition with various aetiologies, each of them causing distinct pathophysiological changes. Understanding these changes is important for effective diagnosis and treatment. Despite its frequent occurrence, the conjunctiva's robust protective mechanisms generally ensure that most cases are self-limiting, allowing the eye to recover fully with appropriate management.

EPIDEMIOLOGY

Conjunctivitis is a commonly encountered condition in ophthalmology clinics throughout the world (Azari and Arabi 2020), a condition often encountered in the primary care setting in the UK (Galloway et al. 2022). There is no significant difference in incidence based on gender, ethnicity or social status; however, the highest rates of diagnosis are observed in children under the age of seven years.

Wilson and Wilson (2021) provide epidemiological data concerning conjunctivitis. Conjunctivitis affects around 2% of the global population. In the United States, about six million people experience the disease annually, accounting for roughly 1% of all primary care visits. In the UK, conjunctivitis is the reason for 1.2–3% of general practitioner visits and affects an estimated 13 out of every 1000 people each year.

Regarding the infectious causes of conjunctivitis, viruses are responsible for about 70% of cases, with bacteria being the next most common cause. The type of microbe causing the infection varies by age. In children, bacteria are responsible for 50–75% of cases, while in adults, viruses are the predominant cause of infection.

Acute infective conjunctivitis accounts for about 1% of all GP consultations in the UK.

Viral conjunctivitis is the most common type of infectious conjunctivitis, responsible for up to 80% of acute conjunctivitis cases. The herpes simplex virus is estimated to cause 1.3–4.8% of acute conjunctivitis cases.

Bacterial conjunctivitis is the second most common cause of infectious conjunctivitis. In children, 50–75% of infective conjunctivitis cases are thought to be due to bacterial infection.

OPHTHALMIA NEONATORUM

- In the UK, the incidence of ophthalmia neonatorum is caused by:

  - *Chlamydia trachomatis* is 6.9 per 100000 live births.

  - *Neisseria gonorrhoeae* is 3.7 per 100000 live births (College of Optometrists 2021).

- An analysis of hospital episode statistics from 2000 to 2011 in England found the incidence rate of hospitalised cases of ophthalmia neonatorum to be 257 per 100000 live births in 2011 (95% CI, 245–269). Marked cyclical fluctuations in incidence were noted over time (the number of cases of ophthalmia neonatorum did not remain constant but instead showed significant patterns of increase and decrease at regular intervals over the observed period), (Dharmasena et al. 2015).

- Viral ophthalmia neonatorum (e.g. due to herpes simplex, adenovirus and enterovirus) is less common.

Conjunctivitis affects different age groups and demonstrates seasonal patterns, especially in allergic cases. Public health measures focus on prevention, early diagnosis and appropriate management to reduce the incidence and transmission of this condition.

RISK FACTORS

Conjunctivitis, while often considered a minor and self-limiting condition, can present various risks depending on its cause and the patient's overall health. Table 5.1 outlines the risks associated with different types of conjunctivitis.

Table 5.1 Risks associated with different types of conjunctivitis

Type of conjunctivitis	Discussion
Viral conjunctivitis	Highly contagious, especially adenoviral conjunctivitis.
	Can lead to outbreaks in schools, workplaces and other communal settings.
	Complications:
	Prolonged inflammation: Can persist for weeks in some cases.
	Secondary bacterial infection: Can develop if the eye is repeatedly rubbed or hygiene is poor.
	Keratitis: In severe cases, the cornea can become involved. This can then lead to keratitis, which may cause vision problems.
Bacterial conjunctivitis	Also highly contagious.
	Can spread through direct contact with infected secretions or contaminated objects.
	Complications:
	Corneal ulceration: Particularly with *Neisseria gonorrhoeae* or *Chlamydia trachomatis* infections.
	Chronicity: If inadequately treated, cases can become chronic.
	Vision impairment: Severe or untreated cases can lead to scarring of the cornea and subsequent vision impairment.
Allergic conjunctivitis	Symptoms and quality of life:
	Persistent itching and discomfort: Can significantly impact a person's daily activities.
	Sleep disturbances: Severe itching and discomfort can lead to poor sleep quality.
	Complications:
	Conjunctival hypertrophy: Chronic allergic conjunctivitis can lead to thickening of the conjunctiva.
	Secondary infections: Excessive rubbing of the eyes can lead to secondary bacterial infections.
Chemical/irritant conjunctivitis	Risks and complications:
	Corneal damage: Depending on the substance, severe irritation can cause corneal damage as well as vision impairment.
	Chronic irritation: Prolonged exposure to irritants (such as chlorine in swimming pools) can lead to chronic conjunctivitis.

Source: Adapted from Azari and Arabi (2020), Bielory et al. (2019) and Wilson and Wilson (2021).

GENERAL RISKS ACROSS ALL TYPES

These can impact on a person's daily life. Highly contagious forms can lead to significant absenteeism from school and work. The redness, swelling and discharge can be problematic due to discomfort and inconvenience.

Misdiagnosis of bacterial conjunctivitis as viral can lead to incorrect treatment and the inappropriate use of antibiotics. A delay in appropriate treatment due to misidentifying allergic conjunctivitis as infectious can delay appropriate anti-allergic treatment.

POPULATIONS AT HIGHER RISK

Conjunctivitis can affect anyone, but there are certain populations who are at higher risk due to various factors such as age, environment and pre-existing conditions.

NEONATES

Ophthalmia neonatorum is a severe form of conjunctivitis caused by bacteria acquired during childbirth. Immediate treatment is crucial to prevent complications such as blindness.

IMMUNOCOMPROMISED INDIVIDUALS

Immunocompromised individuals have weakened immune systems, making them more susceptible to infections, including conjunctivitis. These individuals have a higher risk of severe conjunctival infection. They are more likely to develop complications and require a more intensive form of treatment.

CONTACT LENS WEARERS

People who wear contact lenses are at an increased risk of developing conjunctivitis and other eye infections due to several factors that are related to the use and care of their contact lenses. Increased risk of infection can occur with improper lens hygiene:

- Contact lenses can become contaminated with bacteria or fungi if not handled, cleaned or stored properly. For instance, failing to wash hands before handling lenses, using tap water instead of sterile solution or not cleaning the lenses and storage case regularly can introduce pathogens to the eyes.

- Lenses and storage cases can develop biofilms, which are colonies of bacteria that adhere to surfaces and are resistant to cleaning. This makes infections more likely and harder to treat.

In the context of contact lens wearers, these individuals are more likely to experience infections that spread to the cornea, the clear, dome-shaped surface that covers the front of the eye. There is a higher risk of corneal involvement.

- Contact lenses sit directly on the cornea, the transparent front part of the eye. If lenses are contaminated, the pathogens have direct access to the cornea, increasing the likelihood of infection spreading from the conjunctiva (the membrane covering the white part of the eye) to the cornea.

- Inserting and removing lenses can cause tiny abrasions on the cornea (microtrauma). These small injuries can provide an entry point for bacteria or fungi and as such facilitated the transmission of infection.

Understanding these risks and adopting preventive measures, the impact of conjunctivitis can be minimised and complications can be avoided.

CLINICAL PRESENTATION

Regardless of the underlying cause, any form of inflammation in or around the eye can lead to common symptoms that include increased tearing, discharge and redness due to conjunctival vascular dilation. These symptoms are part of the body's natural inflammatory response to help protect and heal the affected tissues.

The several types of conjunctivitis each have distinct clinical features (see Table 5.2).

Table 5.2 Clinical features associated with conjunctivitis

Type of conjunctivitis	Clinical features
Viral conjunctivitis	Viral conjunctivitis is highly contagious and this is often associated with viral upper respiratory infections. Clinical features: Redness: Diffuse redness of the conjunctiva. Watery discharge: Clear, watery discharge is typical. Tearing: Increased tearing. Itching: Mild to moderate itching. Foreign body sensation: Patients may complain of a feeling of something being in the eye. Swollen eyelids: Mild swelling of the eyelids may occur. Follicles: Small bumps on the conjunctiva, often more pronounced on the lower eyelid. Systemic symptoms: Often this type of conjunctivitis accompanies cold or flu-like symptoms, such as sore throat, fever and runny nose. Unilateral onset: Often starts in one eye and may spread to the other eye.
Bacterial conjunctivitis	Bacterial conjunctivitis is caused by bacterial infections and is also highly contagious. Clinical features: Redness: Marked redness of the conjunctiva may occur. Purulent discharge: Thick, yellow or green discharge that may cause the eyelids to stick together, especially after the person has been asleep. Swollen eyelids: There is more pronounced swelling compared to viral conjunctivitis. Tearing: Increased tearing. Irritation: Mild to moderate discomfort or irritation. Crusting: Crusting of the eyelids and eyelashes. Unilateral or bilateral: Can affect one or both eyes.

(Continued)

Table 5.2 (*Continued*)

Type of conjunctivitis	Clinical features
Allergic conjunctivitis	Allergic conjunctivitis is triggered by allergens such as pollen, dust mites, pet dander and certain chemicals.
	Clinical features:
	Redness: Redness of the conjunctiva.
	Itching: There is intense itching, which is a hallmark symptom.
	Watery discharge: Clear, watery discharge.
	Swollen eyelids: The area around the eyelids becomes enlarged or puffy due to the accumulation of fluid or inflammation.
	Bilateral involvement: Usually affects both eyes simultaneously.
	Seasonal variation: Symptoms may be seasonal (hay fever) or perennial (year-round, due to indoor allergens).
Non-infectious conjunctivitis	This type includes irritative and chemical conjunctivitis that is caused by exposure to irritants or toxic substances.
	Clinical features:
	Redness: Redness of the conjunctiva.
	Discharge: Watery discharge, less commonly purulent (contains or produces pus) unless there is a secondary infection.
	Tearing: Increased tearing.
	Burning or stinging: Sensation of burning or stinging in the eyes.
	Pain: Variable pain. This depends on the severity of the irritant.
	History of exposure: Often associated with a history of exposure to an irritant, such as smoke, chlorine in swimming pools or chemicals (see Box 5.1).
Chronic conjunctivitis	Chronic conjunctivitis persists for more than three weeks and can be due to persistent infection, chronic allergies or underlying eyelid diseases such as blepharitis.
	Clinical features:
	Redness: Persistent redness of the conjunctiva.
	Discharge: There is continuous or recurrent discharge, which may be watery or mucopurulent.
	Irritation: Ongoing irritation or discomfort.
	Eyelid changes: Associated with conditions such as blepharitis or meibomian gland dysfunction (a condition affecting the meibomian glands, located in the eyelids).
	Vision changes: Blurred vision if the cornea is affected.
	Lid crusting: Recurrent crusting of the eyelids, especially upon waking.

Immediate care for patients exposed to chemicals as an act of violence involves rapid assessment, decontamination and stabilisation to prevent further injury and ensure their safety.

The severity of a chemical burn can be minimised if action is taken promptly to remove the chemical and contaminated clothing from contact with the skin or eyes. However, without proper precautions, attempting to assist yourself or others may result in further harm to the victim or cause contact injuries to the person providing help.

Those who witness acid attacks have been issued with advice on how to help victims, as the number of assaults with corrosive substances continues to rise. Victims can be left blind or severely disfigured and the minutes following an attack are critical in helping those who have been affected.

Report, Remove, Rinse guidance from NHS England urges witnesses or victims to **report** the attack by calling 999, carefully **remove** contaminated clothing and immediately **rinse** skin in running water.

NHS England (2017)

Each type of conjunctivitis presents with specific clinical features that guide diagnosis and management. Understanding these features can help those who offer people with conjunctivitis care and support to provide appropriate treatment and advice to minimising discomfort and preventing the spread of infectious forms.

CLINICAL INVESTIGATIONS AND DIAGNOSIS

Conjunctivitis is a diagnosis of exclusion; this means that conjunctivitis is often diagnosed after other potential causes of eye redness and irritation have been ruled out. This approach is taken because there are many conditions that can present with similar symptoms.

Diagnosing conjunctivitis usually involves a combination of history taking, clinical examination and specific diagnostic tests. The goal is to identify the underlying cause, which can be viral, bacterial, allergic or non-infectious.

PATIENT HISTORY

Taking a thorough history is important for diagnosing conjunctivitis and differentiating it from other eye conditions. Azari and Arabi (2020) in their systematic review regarding conjunctivitis, discuss a range of issues to be discussed during the history-taking phase.

Chief Complaint   The initial question to the patient is 'What brings you in today?'

Identify if there are any specific symptoms the person is experiencing. For example:

- Redness

- Itching

- Discharge

- Tearing

- Photophobia

- Pain

- Blurred vision

Symptom Onset and Duration

Onset: 'When did you first notice the symptoms?'
Duration: 'How long have you been experiencing these symptoms?'
Progression: 'Have the symptoms been getting better, worse or staying the same?'

Symptom Characteristics

Redness: 'Is the redness in one eye or both eyes?'
Discharge:

- Type: 'Is the discharge watery, mucoid or purulent?'

- Colour: 'What colour is the discharge?'

- Amount: 'How much discharge do you notice?'

- Sticking: 'Do your eyelids stick together, especially in the morning?'

Itching: 'Do you feel itching in your eyes'?
Tearing: 'Do your eyes water excessively?'
Pain: 'Do you feel any pain in or around your eyes?'
Photophobia: 'Are your eyes sensitive to light?'
Vision changes: 'Have you noticed any changes in your vision?'

Associated Symptoms

Respiratory symptoms: 'Do you have any cold or flu symptoms, such as a sore throat, cough or runny nose?'
Systemic symptoms: 'Do you have a fever or feel generally unwell?'
Lymphadenopathy: 'Have you noticed any swollen glands around your ears or neck?'

Exposure History

Contact with infected individuals: 'Have you been in close contact with anyone who has red or infected eyes recently?'
Recent illness: 'Have you had any recent illnesses or infections?'
Travel history: 'Have you travelled anywhere recently where you might have been exposed to new environments or infectious agents?'

Allergies and Irritants

Allergic history: 'Do you have a history of allergies, such as hay fever or allergic rhinitis?'
Exposure to allergens: 'Have you been exposed to any known allergens, such as pollen, pet dander or dust?'
Irritants: 'Have you been exposed to smoke, chemicals or any other irritants?'

Use of Contact Lenses

Lens type: 'Do you wear contact lenses? If so, what type (soft, hard, daily disposables, extended wear)?'
Hygiene: 'How do you care for and clean your contact lenses?'
Wearing schedule: 'How long do you wear your contact lenses each day? Do you sleep in them?'

Previous Eye Conditions and Treatments

History of conjunctivitis: 'Have you had conjunctivitis or any other eye infections before?'

Chronic eye conditions: 'Do you have any chronic eye conditions, such as dry eye syndrome (also known as dry eye disease or keratoconjunctivitis sicca, where the eyes do not produce enough tears or the tears evaporate too quickly, leading to dryness, discomfort and potential damage to the ocular surface) or blepharitis?'

Previous treatments: 'Have you used any eye drops or ointments recently? If so, what were they and did they help?'

Medical History

Chronic illnesses: 'Do you have any chronic illnesses, such as diabetes or autoimmune diseases?'

Medications: 'What medications are you currently taking, including over-the-counter drugs and supplements?'

Social and Occupational History

Occupation: 'Do you have a job? If so, what type of work do you do? Are you exposed to any irritants or allergens at work?'

Hobbies and activities: 'Do you engage in activities that might expose your eyes to irritants, such as swimming or using makeup?'

Taking a comprehensive history involves detailed questioning about the onset, duration and characteristics of symptoms, associated systemic symptoms, exposure history and personal and medical background. This information helps differentiate between viral, bacterial, allergic and non-infectious causes of conjunctivitis and guides appropriate diagnostic and therapeutic measures.

CLINICAL EXAMINATION

A detailed physical examination is essential to diagnose conjunctivitis accurately and to differentiate it from other ocular conditions. It is essential that local policies and procedures related to consent, the provision of a chaperone and infection prevention and control requirements are adhered to.

A visual inspection is undertaken. Evaluation of the extent and distribution of redness is determined. Conjunctival redness is typically diffuse and involves the palpebral (lining the eyelids) and bulbar (covering the eyeball) conjunctiva. The patient's eyelid is assessed for conjunctival swelling (chemosis). Significant swelling may suggest a more severe infection or allergic reaction.

The type of discharge is assessed to determine whether it is watery, mucoid or purulent. Watery discharge is common in viral and allergic conjunctivitis, whereas purulent discharge suggests a bacterial infection. The quantity of discharge is noted and whether it is persistent or intermittent. Ascertain if the discharge is in one or both eyes: conjunctivitis can start in one eye and spread to the other. Bilateral involvement is more common in viral and allergic conjunctivitis.

Eyelid Examination The patient is observed for signs of eyelid oedema, which can be a sign of severe allergic reactions or infection. Observation is made for crusting, especially in bacterial conjunctivitis, where purulent discharge can cause the eyelids to stick together.

Checks are made for any lesions, ulcers or vesicles on the eyelids, which might indicate herpetic infections (herpes simplex virus).

Conjunctival Evaluation The degree of redness and whether it is localised or diffuse is assessed. Diffuse redness is typical of conjunctivitis, while sectoral redness (this refers to a specific pattern of redness in the eye that can help differentiate between different types of eye conditions) may suggest episcleritis. Small, dome-shaped lymphoid structures typically seen in viral conjunctivitis and chlamydial infections may be observed. They appear as small, white or pale yellow bumps. Elevated lesions with a red, vascular centre are commonly seen in allergic conjunctivitis and bacterial conjunctivitis. They resemble cobblestone patterns, especially under the upper eyelid. Pseudomembranes can be seen in severe viral or bacterial infections. Membranes can be peeled away from the conjunctiva, while true membranes are firmly adherent and may bleed when removed. Pseudomembranes and membranes are structures that can form on the conjunctiva in certain types of conjunctivitis and other inflammatory eye conditions. They are indicators of more severe or advanced disease and can help in differentiating between different causes of conjunctivitis.

Corneal Involvement The cornea is checked for clarity. Any haziness or opacification could indicate keratitis or other serious conditions. Signs of inflammation or infection extending to the cornea are known as corneal infiltrates. The patient is assessed for corneal ulcers, which are serious and require immediate attention.

Lymphadenopathy Preauricular lymph nodes are palpated for signs of enlargement (these lymph nodes are located in front of the ears, near the area where the ear connects to the side of the head). Enlarged and tender preauricular nodes are often associated with viral conjunctivitis, particularly adenoviral infections. The submandibular lymph nodes are also checked. The submandibular lymph nodes also known as submaxillary lymph nodes are assessed; a group of lymph nodes located beneath the lower jaw (mandible) on either side of the neck.

INVESTIGATIONS

A range of investigations may be undertaken to confirm or contest a diagnosis of conjunctivitis (see Table 5.3). Local policy and procedure along with national guidelines will guide the type(s) of investigation to be carried out.

Table 5.3 Investigations used in a diagnosis of conjunctivitis

Investigation	Discussion
Slit-lamp examination	Provides a detailed view of the anterior segment of the eye.
	Helps in assessing the conjunctiva, cornea and anterior chamber for inflammation, foreign bodies or other abnormalities.
Conjunctival swab and culture	A swab is taken from the conjunctival sac to identify bacterial, viral or fungal pathogens.
	Culture and sensitivity tests help in identifying the causative organism and determining appropriate antibiotic treatment in bacterial cases.
Polymerase chain reaction testing	Highly sensitive and specific test for detecting viral pathogens, particularly adenovirus, which is a common cause of viral conjunctivitis.
	Useful in outbreaks or when the diagnosis is uncertain.

Investigation	Discussion
Allergy testing	Skin prick tests or specific IgE blood tests may be conducted if allergic conjunctivitis is suspected.
	Identifies specific allergens responsible for the condition.
Tear film and ocular surface tests	Tear break-up time (TBUT): Measures tear film stability. A short TBUT can indicate dry eye, which can coexist with or mimic conjunctivitis.
	Schirmer test: Measures tear production to assess for dry eye syndrome.
	Ocular surface staining: Uses dyes such as fluorescein to highlight damage or irregularities on the ocular surface.
Blood tests	In cases of suspected systemic infection or autoimmune disease, blood tests might be required.
	Full blood count and inflammatory markers (such as C-reactive protein) can provide information about the systemic response to infection or inflammation.

Source: Adapted from Wilson and Wilson (2021); Borooah and Tint (2023).

The clinical investigation for diagnosing conjunctivitis involves a thorough patient history and physical examination, supplemented by specific tests such as conjunctival swabs, PCR testing, allergy testing and tear film assessment. These investigations help in identifying the underlying cause of conjunctivitis and guiding appropriate treatment. Accurate diagnosis is essential for effective management and to prevent complications or the spread of infectious forms of conjunctivitis.

MANAGEMENT

The management of conjunctivitis varies depending on the underlying cause, whether it is bacterial, viral, allergic or due to other factors.

BACTERIAL CONJUNCTIVITIS

TOPICAL ANTIBIOTICS

- Common options include erythromycin ointment, sulfacetamide drops, polymyxin B/trimethoprim drops or fluoroquinolone drops.

- Typically applied three to four times a day for 7–10 days.

HYGIENE MEASURES

- Regular hand washing.

- Avoiding touching or rubbing the eyes.

- Clearing away discharge with a clean, damp cloth.

- Contact lens users should discontinue use of lenses during treatment and consider replacing lenses and lens cases.

While antibiotic treatment can speed up recovery and reduce transmission risk, it should be noted that many cases of bacterial conjunctivitis are self-limiting.

VIRAL CONJUNCTIVITIS

SUPPORTIVE CARE

- Artificial tears can be used to alleviate dryness and irritation.
- Cold compresses to reduce swelling and discomfort.

HYGIENE MEASURES

- Avoid sharing towels, pillows or other personal items.
- Frequent hand washing.
- Avoiding touching the eyes.

ANTIVIRAL MEDICATIONS

Generally, these are not required unless the infection is caused by herpes simplex virus, where antiviral therapy (e.g. acyclovir) might be indicated (Galloway et al. 2022).

Viral conjunctivitis is highly contagious. Symptoms will usually resolve within one to two weeks without specific treatment.

ALLERGIC CONJUNCTIVITIS

Identify and minimise exposure to allergens (e.g. pollen, dust mites, pet dander).

MEDICATIONS

- Antihistamine eye drops: Ketotifen, olopatadine or azelastine.
- Mast cell stabilisers (a class of medications used to manage allergic conjunctivitis and other allergic conditions).
- Combined antihistamine/mast cell stabilisers: Provide immediate and long-term relief.
- Oral antihistamines: Used for systemic allergy control (e.g. cetirizine, loratadine).
- Cold compresses can be used to relieve itching and swelling.

Persistent cases may require referral to an allergist for further evaluation and management.

CHEMICAL CONJUNCTIVITIS

- Immediate irrigation: Flush the eyes with copious amounts of water or saline for at least 15–30 minutes.
- Emergency care: Seek immediate medical attention.

- Symptomatic treatment: Use of artificial tears and cold compresses.

Prompt and thorough irrigation is critical to minimise damage. Follow-up care with an ophthalmologist may be necessary.

FURTHER CONSIDERATIONS

Accurate diagnosis is crucial to ensure appropriate treatment with an assessment of the type and severity of conjunctivitis. Patient education is key to prevent transmission and complications. Those with bacterial or viral conjunctivitis should stay home to reduce the spread until symptoms improve or, in the case of bacterial conjunctivitis, after 24 hours of antibiotic treatment.

Management of conjunctivitis involves identifying the underlying cause and providing appropriate treatment, whether it be antibiotics for bacterial infections, supportive care for viral infections, allergy management for allergic conjunctivitis or immediate irrigation for chemical exposures. Effective hygiene practices and patient education are key components to prevent the transmission and ensure effective management.

HEALTH TEACHING

Health teaching for patients with conjunctivitis is important in ensuring effective management, prevent transmission and promote recovery. Table 5.4 provides the key areas to focus on.

Health teaching for people with conjunctivitis should cover understanding the type of conjunctivitis, infection control, proper medication use, symptom management, recognising complications, lifestyle modifications and general eye care. Providing comprehensive education helps patients manage their condition effectively, reduce the risk of transmission and promote quicker recovery.

Table 5.4 Key areas to focus on with regards to the health teaching needs of people with conjunctivitis

Health teaching need	Discussion
Understanding conjunctivitis	Types of conjunctivitis: Offer patients information about the different types of conjunctivitis – bacterial, viral, allergic and chemical. Each type has distinct causes, symptoms and treatments.
	Bacterial: Typically involves purulent discharge and may affect one or both eyes.
	Viral: Often associated with watery discharge and preauricular lymphadenopathy.
	Allergic: Characterised by itching, redness and watery discharge, often bilateral.
	Chemical: Caused by exposure to irritants and requires immediate irrigation.
Infection prevention and control	Hand hygiene: Emphasise the importance of frequent hand washing with soap and water to prevent the spread of infection.
	Avoid touching eyes: Advise against touching or rubbing the eyes to reduce irritation and prevent spreading organisms.
	Personal items: Do not share personal items such as towels, washcloths, pillows or cosmetics.
	Contact lens hygiene: For contact lens wearers, discontinue lens use until the infection clears. Clean the lenses and cases thoroughly before resuming use.

(Continued)

Table 5.4   (*Continued*)

Health teaching need	Discussion
Use of medication	Antibiotic eye drops/ointments: For bacterial conjunctivitis, advise the patient on the correct application technique and the importance of completing the full course of antibiotics even if symptoms improve.
	Antihistamine or mast cell stabiliser drops: For allergic conjunctivitis, explain the need for regular use to prevent symptoms.
	Lubricating drops: For comfort in viral and allergic conjunctivitis, recommend preservative-free artificial tears.
Symptom management	Cold compresses: Can reduce swelling and discomfort, particularly for allergic and viral conjunctivitis.
	Warm compresses: For bacterial conjunctivitis to help loosen crusts on the eyelids.
	Pain relief: Over-the-counter pain relievers, for example, paracetamol or ibuprofen, can be used for discomfort.
Recognising complications	Worsening symptoms: Advise patients to seek medical attention if symptoms worsen, do not improve with treatment or if they experience severe pain, light sensitivity or vision changes.
	Follow-up care: Encourage follow-up visits to monitor progress, especially for bacterial and severe viral conjunctivitis.
Lifestyle and environmental modifications	Avoid allergens: For allergic conjunctivitis, identify and minimise exposure to known allergens such as pollen, dust or pet dander.
	Work and school attendance: Advise on the appropriate duration to stay home from work or school to prevent spreading infectious conjunctivitis. Typically, patients can return once symptoms improve or after 24 hours of antibiotic treatment for bacterial conjunctivitis.
General eye care	Avoid eye makeup: During an active infection, avoid using eye makeup to prevent further irritation and contamination.
	Sunglasses: Wearing sunglasses can help reduce light sensitivity and protect the eyes from irritants.

Source: Adapted from Sanderson (2019).

CONCLUSION

Conjunctivitis encompasses a range of inflammatory conditions of the conjunctiva, characterised by redness, irritation, discharge and varying degrees of discomfort. It can be classified into bacterial, viral, allergic and chemical types, each with distinct aetiologies and management strategies.

Bacterial conjunctivitis, often marked by purulent discharge, typically responds well to topical antibiotics, while viral conjunctivitis, frequently associated with watery discharge and preauricular lymphadenopathy, usually requires supportive care. Allergic conjunctivitis, driven by allergens, benefits from antihistamines, mast cell stabilisers and avoiding known triggers. Chemical conjunctivitis demands immediate irrigation and emergency care to prevent ocular damage.

Effective management of conjunctivitis hinges on accurate diagnosis, appropriate treatment and comprehensive patient education. Ensuring patients understand the nature of their condition, the importance of hygiene and the correct use of medications is crucial for recovery and preventing transmission, particularly in infectious cases.

Those who offer care and support to people with conjunctivitis play a pivotal role in guiding patients through the nuances of conjunctivitis, from recognising symptoms to implementing preventive measures and understanding when to seek further medical attention. Integrating these elements can help to enhance patient outcomes and mitigate the public health impact of this common but often disruptive condition.

Conjunctivitis is a multifaceted condition requiring a nuanced approach tailored to its various forms. Through diligent diagnosis, targeted treatment and robust patient education, the condition can be effectively managed and mitigate the impacts of conjunctivitis, ensuring better health and comfort for affected individuals.

GLOSSARY OF TERMS

Allergic conjunctivitis: Inflammation of the conjunctiva caused by allergens such as pollen, dust mites or pet dander, characterised by itching, redness and watery discharge.

Antihistamines: Medications that block histamine receptors to reduce allergic symptoms, including those associated with allergic conjunctivitis.

Artificial tears: Lubricating eye drops used to relieve dryness and irritation in various types of conjunctivitis, especially viral and allergic.

Bacterial conjunctivitis: A type of conjunctivitis caused by bacterial infection, characterised by purulent discharge, redness and irritation.

Chemical conjunctivitis: Inflammation of the conjunctiva caused by exposure to irritants or chemicals, requiring immediate irrigation to prevent damage.

Conjunctiva: The thin, transparent tissue covering the white part of the eye (sclera) and the inner surface of the eyelids.

Corticosteroids: Anti-inflammatory medications sometimes used in severe cases of allergic conjunctivitis to reduce inflammation.

Cromolyn sodium: A mast cell stabiliser used in eye drops to prevent allergic conjunctivitis symptoms by inhibiting the release of histamine.

Discharge: Fluid released from the eyes, which can be watery, mucoid or purulent, depending on the type of conjunctivitis.

Follicles: Small, dome-shaped nodules on the conjunctiva, often seen in viral conjunctivitis.

Histamine: A chemical released during allergic reactions that causes symptoms such as itching, redness and swelling in allergic conjunctivitis.

Infectious conjunctivitis: Conjunctivitis caused by bacterial or viral infections, characterised by symptoms such as redness, discharge and contagiousness.

Lymphadenopathy: Swelling of the lymph nodes, which can occur in viral conjunctivitis, particularly the preauricular lymph nodes.

Mast cell stabilisers: Medications that prevent the release of histamine and other chemicals from mast cells, used to treat allergic conjunctivitis.

Meibomian gland dysfunction: A condition where the oil glands in the eyelids do not function properly, potentially leading to dry eyes and secondary conjunctivitis.

Papillae: Raised, flat-topped areas on the conjunctiva, often seen in allergic conjunctivitis.

Preauricular lymph nodes: Lymph nodes located in front of the ears, which can become enlarged in viral conjunctivitis.

Pseudomembranes/membranes: Layers of inflammatory cells and fibrin that can form on the conjunctiva in severe infections.

Purulent: Describing a type of discharge that is thick and yellow or green, indicative of bacterial conjunctivitis.

Topical antibiotics: Medications applied directly to the eye to treat bacterial conjunctivitis.

Viral conjunctivitis: Inflammation of the conjunctiva caused by viral infections, characterised by watery discharge, redness and often accompanied by cold-like symptoms.

MULTIPLE CHOICE QUESTIONS

1. Which type of conjunctivitis is characterised by purulent discharge?
   a) Viral conjunctivitis
   b) Allergic conjunctivitis
   c) Bacterial conjunctivitis
   d) Chemical conjunctivitis

2. What is the first line of treatment for bacterial conjunctivitis?
   a) Antiviral medication
   b) Antihistamines
   c) Topical antibiotics
   d) Corticosteroids

3. Which of the following symptoms is most commonly associated with viral conjunctivitis?
   a) Purulent discharge
   b) Itching
   c) Watery discharge
   d) Severe pain

4. Which type of conjunctivitis is often associated with hay fever?
   a) Bacterial conjunctivitis
   b) Viral conjunctivitis
   c) Allergic conjunctivitis
   d) Chemical conjunctivitis

5. What is a common cause of chemical conjunctivitis?
   a) Bacterial infection
   b) Viral infection
   c) Exposure to irritants
   d) Allergens

6. Which medication is a mast cell stabiliser used for treating allergic conjunctivitis?
   a) Erythromycin
   b) Olopatadine
   c) Cromolyn sodium
   d) Acyclovir

7. What is the main preventive measure for the spread of viral conjunctivitis?
   a) Using antibiotics
   b) Avoiding allergens
   c) Frequent hand washing
   d) Wearing sunglasses

8. What is the recommended action immediately after exposure to a chemical irritant in the eye?
   a) Apply antibiotic ointment
   b) Flush the eye with water or saline
   c) Use antihistamine drops
   d) Take oral antihistamines

9. Which lymph nodes are often enlarged in viral conjunctivitis?
   a) Submandibular nodes
   b) Preauricular lymph nodes
   c) Cervical lymph nodes
   d) Axillary lymph nodes

10. Which type of conjunctivitis is most likely to be associated with a sore throat and common cold symptoms?
   a) Bacterial conjunctivitis
   b) Viral conjunctivitis
   c) Allergic conjunctivitis
   d) Chemical conjunctivitis

REFERENCES

Azari, A A. and Arabi, A. (2020). Conjunctivitis: a systematic review. *Journal of Ophthalmic Vision Research* 15 (3): 372–395.

Bielory, L., Delgado, L., Katelaris, C.H. et al. (2019). Diagnosis and management of allergic conjunctivitis. *Annal of Allergy, Asthma and Immunology* 124 (2): 118–134. doi: 10.1016/j.anai.2019.11.014.

Borooah, S. and Tint, N.L. (2023). The visual system (Chapter 8). In: *Macleod's Clinical Examination*, 15e (eds. A. R. Dover, J. A. Innes, and K. Fairhurst). London: Elsevier.

College of Optometrists (2021). Conjunctivitis, chlamydial. https://www.college-optometrists.org/clinical-guidance/clinical-management-guidelines/conjunctivitis_chlamydial_adultinclusionconjunctiv (accessed July 2024).

Dharmasena, A., Hall, N., Goldacre, R. et al. (2015). Time trends in ophthalmia neonatorum and dacryocystitis of the newborn in England, 2000–2011: database study. *Sexually Transmitted Infections* 91 (5): 342–345.

Galloway, N.R., Amoaku, W.M., Galloway, P.H. et al. (2022). *Common Eye Diseases and their Management*, 5e. London: Springer.

NHS England (2017). New help for 'acid attack' victims following recent rise in demand for NHS help. https://www.england.nhs.uk/2017/08/new-help-for-acid-attack-victims-following-recent-rise-in-demand-for-nhs-help/ (accessed July 2024).

Sanderson, A. (2019). Nursing patients with disorders of the eye and sight impairment. In: *Alexanders's Nursing Practice*, 6e (ed. I. Peate). London: Elsevier.

Wilson, M. and Wilson, P.J.K. (2021). Conjunctivitis (Chapter 19). In: *Close Encounters of the Microbial Kind* (eds. M. Wilson and P.J.K. Wilson). doi: 10.1007/978-3-030-56978-5_19.

CHAPTER 6

Age-related Macular Degeneration

MACULAR DEGENERATION

Macular degeneration is a condition that affects the central part of the retina, known as the macula, leading to vision loss. The most common type is age-related macular degeneration (AMD), which can be further classified into two main forms: dry (atrophic) AMD and wet (neovascular or exudative) AMD. Additionally, there are other less common types of macular degeneration, each with distinct characteristics and causes.

OTHER TYPES OF MACULAR DEGENERATION

Juvenile Macular Degeneration (Stargardt Disease) Stargardt disease is a genetic form of macular degeneration that typically affects children and young adults. A change in a particular gene can cause waste material called lipofuscin to build-up in a part of the eye called the retinal pigment epithelium (RPE). This build-up causes damage to the cells in the macula, which are responsible for clear central vision, leading to vision problems. Symptoms include central vision loss at a young age, making activities such as reading and face recognition difficult (Royal National Institute of Blind People 2024).

Myopic Macular Degeneration This type of macular degeneration occurs in individuals with high myopia (severe near-sightedness). It is due to the stretching and thinning of the retina, which can lead to degenerative changes in the macula. Similar to wet AMD, myopic macular degeneration can involve choroidal neovascularisation. This is the growth of abnormal blood vessels in the layer of the eye called the choroid. These new blood vessels can leak blood and fluid into the retina, leading to vision problems. Choroidal neovascularisation is often associated with conditions such as AMD. Patients often experience central vision loss and visual distortions.

Macular Degeneration Secondary to Other Conditions Central serous chorioretinopathy is a condition that involves fluid accumulation under the retina, causing a detachment of the RPE and leading to sudden blurred or distorted central vision. A genetic disorder (called Best disease), which usually presents in childhood or adolescence, is characterised by the accumulation of lipofuscin-like material in the macula and variable central vision loss (Royal National Institute of Blind People 2023a). A group of inherited disorders affecting both cones and rods (called cone–rod dystrophy) leads to central vision loss, night blindness and peripheral vision loss.

Macular degeneration encompasses a variety of conditions that lead to the deterioration of the macula, which can often result in the person experiencing significant central vision loss. The most common type, AMD, includes dry and wet forms, each with distinct pathophysiological mechanisms and clinical features. Other types of macular degeneration,

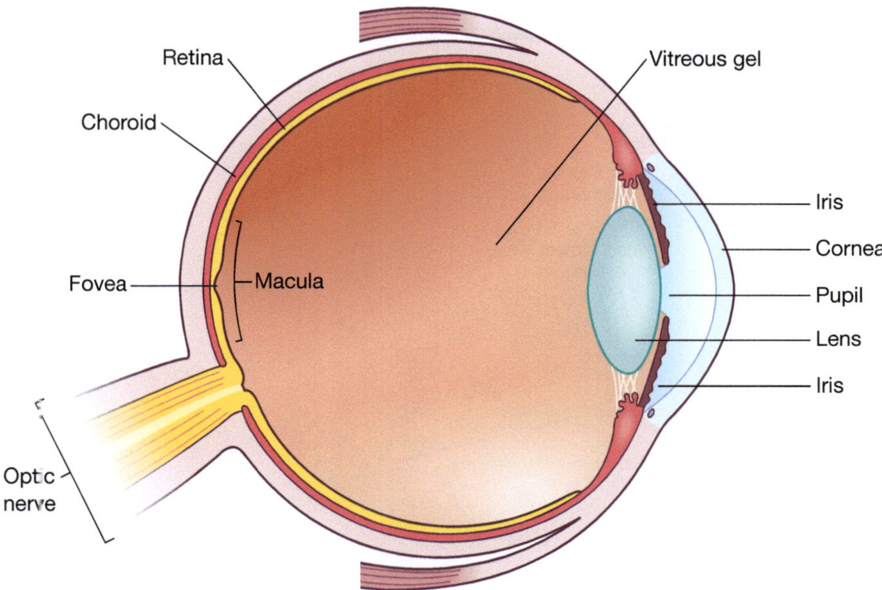

FIGURE 6.1   The eye showing the position of the macula

such as juvenile macular degeneration (Stargardt disease), myopic macular degeneration and those secondary to other conditions, including central serous chorioretinopathy and Best disease, further illustrate the diversity of this group of disorders. Understanding the different types of macular degeneration is crucial for accurate diagnosis, effective management and the development of targeted treatments.

PATHOPHYSIOLOGICAL CHANGES ASSOCIATED WITH AGE-RELATED MACULAR DEGENERATION

Age-related macular degeneration involves a number of pathophysiological changes that primarily affect the macula (see Figure 6.1), the central part of the retina responsible for sharp, detailed vision.

Figure 6.2 demonstrates a normal macula and a degenerated macular.

There are two different forms of macular degeneration that can occur. The American Academy of Ophthalmology (2019) and Royal College of Ophthalmologists (2024), for example, discuss the pathophysiological changes associated with AMD.

DRY (NON-EXUDATIVE OR ATROPHIC)

Dry AMD is the most common form of AMD, representing the initial stage of the disease in the majority of cases. These are the pathophysiological changes associated with dry AMD.

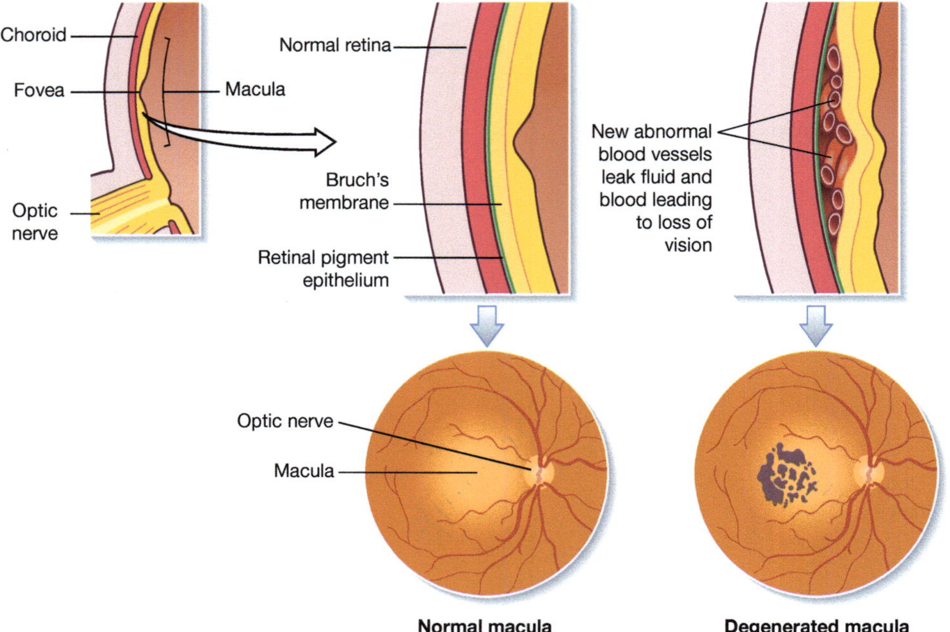

FIGURE 6.2 Normal macula and degenerated macula

RETINAL PIGMENT EPITHELIUM CHANGES

- Role of RPE: The RPE is a layer of cells that are located between the retina and the choroid. It plays a critical role in maintaining the health of photoreceptors (rods and cones) by recycling visual pigments, phagocytising cellular debris and providing essential nutrients.

- Dysfunction: In dry AMD, the RPE becomes less efficient at performing these functions. This dysfunction can lead to the gradual death of RPE cells, impacting the photoreceptors directly above them.

DRUSEN FORMATION

- Accumulation: Drusen are yellowish deposits that form between the RPE and the underlying choroid. They are composed of lipids, proteins and cellular debris.

- Effect: Drusen interfere with the exchange of nutrients and waste products between the RPE and the choroid. Their presence indicates stress and damage to the RPE. Drusen can be classified into soft drusen (larger and more irregular) and hard drusen (smaller and well-defined).

CHORIORETINAL ATROPHY (ALSO CALLED GEOGRAPHIC ATROPHY)

- Progression: As dry AMD progresses, areas of the RPE and photoreceptors undergo atrophy, leading to geographic atrophy. This represents a significant loss of tissue in the macular region.

- Geographic atrophy: This is characterised by well-defined areas where both RPE and photoreceptors are lost. These atrophic areas appear as dark or light spots on imaging studies and are associated with a gradual loss of central vision.

ABSENCE OF KEY FEATURES IN DRY AGE-RELATED MACULAR DEGENERATION

- No elevated macular scar: Unlike wet AMD, dry AMD does not involve the formation of elevated scar tissue that is known as a disciform scar.

- No oedema: There is no swelling or fluid accumulation in the retina, which differentiates dry AMD from the wet form.

- No haemorrhage: Dry AMD does not involve bleeding within the retina or the subretinal space.

- No exudation: There is no leakage of fluid or proteins from abnormal blood vessels, which is characteristic of wet AMD.

INFLAMMATORY AND OXIDATIVE STRESS

Inflammatory and oxidative stress refer to damage caused by chronic inflammation and harmful molecules known as reactive oxygen species (ROS). This damage contributes to diseases such as AMD, where it harms the cells in the eye, leading to vision problems.

- Oxidative damage: Oxidative stress causes cell damage and drusen formation. Ageing and environmental factors such as smoking and sunlight exposure exacerbate this oxidative stress.

- Inflammatory response: Chronic low-grade inflammation can further damage the RPE and contribute to the progression of dry AMD.

Dry AMD begins with changes to the RPE, leading to drusen formation and, in more advanced stages, geographic atrophy. Unlike wet AMD, dry AMD does not feature abnormal blood vessel growth, macular scarring, oedema or haemorrhage. Understanding these pathophysiological changes is crucial for diagnosing, monitoring and managing dry AMD, with a focus on preserving vision and preventing progression to more severe forms of the disease.

WET (NEOVASCULAR OR EXUDATIVE) AGE-RELATED MACULAR DEGENERATION

Wet AMD is a less common but more severe form of AMD, responsible for the majority of significant vision loss associated with the disease. These are the pathophysiological changes associated with wet AMD.

CHOROIDAL NEOVASCULARISATION

- Abnormal blood vessel growth: Wet AMD occurs when new, abnormal blood vessels develop under the retina, specifically originating from the choroid layer. This process is known as choroidal neovascularisation.

- Stimuli for choroidal neovascularisation: Factors such as hypoxia (lack of oxygen) and inflammation stimulate the production of growth factors, notably vascular endothelial growth factor, which promotes the growth of these abnormal blood vessels.

LOCALISED MACULAR OEDEMA AND HAEMORRHAGE

- Leakage and swelling: The newly formed blood vessels in choroidal neovascularisation are fragile and prone to leaking blood and fluid. This leakage leads to localised macular oedema, causing swelling and disrupting the normal architecture of the retina.

- Haemorrhage: The fragile nature of these vessels also means they can easily bleed, leading to haemorrhages under the retina. This can cause acute vision changes and further damage the retinal structure.

RETINAL PIGMENT EPITHELIAL DETACHMENT

- Elevation of the macula: The fluid and blood leakage can cause a localised detachment of the RPE from the underlying tissue. This detachment elevates an area of the macula, and in so doing, it impairs its function.

- Impact on vision: The elevation and detachment of the RPE and overlying retina disrupt the precise alignment and functioning of the photoreceptors, leading to distorted or blurred vision.

FORMATION OF DISCIFORM SCAR

- Chronic damage: If left untreated, the continuous leakage and bleeding from the abnormal vessels lead to the formation of fibrovascular tissue or scar tissue, beneath the macula. This is referred to as a disciform scar.

- Permanent vision loss: The disciform scar causes permanent damage to the macular region, resulting in severe and irreversible central vision loss. The scar tissue disrupts the normal retinal structure and function, leading to significant visual impairment.

OXIDATIVE STRESS AND INFLAMMATION

- Oxidative damage: Similar to dry AMD, oxidative stress plays a critical role in the pathogenesis of wet AMD. ROS causes damage to retinal cells, promoting an environment conducive to choroidal neovascularisation.

- Inflammatory processes: Chronic inflammation contributes to the pathogenesis and progression of wet AMD. Inflammatory cells and cytokines further damage the RPE and surrounding tissues, exacerbating the growth of abnormal vessels.

GENETIC AND ENVIRONMENTAL FACTORS

- Genetic predisposition: Genetic variations, particularly in genes related to the complement system and inflammatory pathways, increase the risk of developing wet AMD.

- Environmental influences: Factors such as smoking, poor diet and excessive sunlight exposure can increase oxidative stress and inflammation, contributing to the development and progression of wet AMD.

Wet AMD is characterised by the abnormal growth of blood vessels (choroidal neovascularisation) under the retina, leading to macular oedema, haemorrhage and eventual formation of scar tissue. Although it affects a smaller percentage of individuals with AMD, it is responsible for the majority of severe vision loss due to the destructive nature of the abnormal vessels and subsequent scarring. Understanding these pathophysiological changes is crucial for the early detection, treatment and management of wet AMD, aiming to preserve vision and prevent irreversible damage.

EPIDEMIOLOGY

The Royal College of Ophthalmologists (2024) in their commissioning guidance provide epidemiological data regarding AMD. The global prevalence of AMD is expected to rise from an estimated 196 million (95% CrI, 140–261) in 2020 to 288 million (95% CrI, 205–399) by 2040. AMD is a common cause of visual impairment among the elderly. Due to longer life expectancies and an ageing population worldwide, early diagnosis and timely management of treatable AMD are crucial to reducing the number of people suffering from avoidable irreversible vision loss. In the UK, it was estimated that in 2012, there were 513 000 cases of late AMD, including 276 000 cases of geographic atrophy and 263 000 cases of neovascular AMD. When these figures are adjusted using updated five-yearly UK population estimates published by the United Nations, the prevalence in 2020 is estimated to be 645 000 cases of late AMD, 354 000 cases of geographic atrophy and 339 000 cases of neovascular AMD. From 2013 to 2050, the proportion of sight loss and blindness from AMD is projected to increase from 23.1 to 29.7%, more than doubling from 445 809 (363 900–532 800) people to 1.23 million (1.01–1.47 million) people. Analysis of certificates of visual impairment indicates that approximately 50% of people registered as sight impaired or severely sight impaired are due to macular and posterior pole degeneration. The incidence in 2020 is estimated to be 83 000 cases of late AMD, 51 000 cases of geographic atrophy and 46 000 cases of neovascular AMD. Increasing age, white ethnicity and smoking are significant risk factors that influence the incidence of AMD.

There are gender differences associated with AMD, and the condition is higher in women. Women are more likely to develop AMD than men (National Institute for Health and Care Excellence [NICE] 2018). This difference is partly due to the longer life expectancy of women, which increases their exposure to risk factors over time. Ethnic variations also exist. AMD is more common in Caucasians compared to other ethnic groups (Royal College of Ophthalmologists 2024).

Age-related macular degeneration is a prevalent condition among older adults in the UK, with increasing prevalence correlating with advancing age. Women and individuals of Caucasian ethnicity are more commonly affected. Socioeconomic status, smoking, diet and other lifestyle factors play significant roles in the epidemiology of AMD. With the ageing population, the burden of AMD is expected to grow, highlighting the need for effective prevention, early detection and management strategies.

RISK FACTORS

Age-related macular degeneration is a complex condition that is influenced by a variety of genetic, environmental and lifestyle factors. Understanding these risk factors is crucial for those who offer people with the condition care and support to prevent complications and manage the illness. Table 6.1 outlines the risk factors associated with AMD.

Table 6.1 Risk factors associated with age-related macular degeneration (AMD)

Risk factors	Discussion
Age	The likelihood of developing AMD increases significantly with age. Age is the primary risk factor. It is rare in individuals under 50 years but becomes more common in those over 60 years, with prevalence rising sharply in people aged 70 years and older.
Genetics	Family history: A family history of AMD significantly increases the risk, suggesting a strong genetic component.
	Specific genes: Variations in certain genes have been linked to a higher risk of AMD. These genes are involved in inflammatory and immune responses.
Ethnicity	AMD is more prevalent among people of Caucasian descent compared to other ethnic groups. The reasons are not fully understood but may relate to genetic and environmental factors.
Smoking	Smoking doubles the risk of developing AMD. The harmful effects of smoking include increased oxidative stress and inflammation, which contribute to retinal damage.
Diet and nutrition	A diet low in antioxidants may increase the risk of AMD. These nutrients help protect the retina from oxidative damage.
	Low intake of omega-3 fatty acids, which are found in fish and some plant oils, is associated with a higher risk of AMD.
Cardiovascular health	Hypertension is associated with an increased risk of AMD, possibly due to its impact on blood flow to the retina.
	The build-up of fatty deposits in the arteries (atherosclerosis) can restrict blood flow to the eyes, increasing the risk of AMD.
Obesity	Higher Body Mass Index is linked to a greater risk of AMD, likely due to associated metabolic and cardiovascular issues.
Sunlight exposure	Prolonged exposure to UV and blue light may increase the risk of AMD. Wearing sunglasses that block UV light can help mitigate this risk.
Gender	Women are slightly more likely to develop AMD than men, which may be partly due to their longer life expectancy.
Alcohol consumption	High alcohol intake is associated with an increased risk of AMD, possibly due to its oxidative effects and impact on nutrient absorption.

Source: Adapted from NICE (2018); American Academy of Ophthalmology (2019).

The presence of AMD in the other eye is also seen as another risk factor. AMD is influenced by a combination of age, genetic predisposition and modifiable lifestyle factors. While some risk factors, such as age and genetics, are beyond control, others – such as smoking cessation, maintaining a healthy diet, managing cardiovascular health and protecting the eyes from excessive sunlight exposure – can help reduce the risk of developing AMD. Understanding these risk factors can guide preventive strategies and inform individuals at higher risk of appropriate lifestyle modifications to preserve their vision.

CLINICAL PRESENTATION

Age-related macular degeneration and its clinical presentation varies depending on whether the AMD is dry (atrophic) or wet (neovascular). Understanding these presentations is crucial for early diagnosis and management.

DRY AGE-RELATED MACULAR DEGENERATION (ATROPHIC)

Dry AMD progresses more slowly and is the more common form, accounting for about 85–90% of AMD cases. The clinical features include:

EARLY STAGES

Drusen: Small yellow deposits called drusen accumulate between the retina and the underlying choroid. Drusen are often detected during routine eye examinations before there are any noticeable vision changes occurring. They are one of the earliest signs of dry AMD.

Mild vision changes: Patients might notice that there is a slight blurring or distortion in central vision. This may manifest as difficulty in reading small print or recognising faces (Sanderson 2021).

INTERMEDIATE STAGES

Increased drusen: As AMD progresses, the number and size of drusen increases. This can be observed during examination of the eyes.

Pigment changes: The RPE, which provides nourishment to the retina, may start to show pigmentary changes. These changes can cause dark or light spots in vision.

ADVANCED STAGES

Geographic atrophy: In advanced dry AMD, there is a gradual breakdown of the RPE and loss of photoreceptors, leading to areas of atrophy. These areas appear as patches of missing retina and cause blind spots (scotomas) in central vision.

Significant vision loss: Central vision deteriorates more noticeably, making it difficult to perform tasks that require sharp vision, such as reading and driving. However, peripheral vision remains intact.

WET AGE-RELATED MACULAR DEGENERATION (NEOVASCULAR OR EXUDATIVE)

Wet AMD progresses more rapidly and is less common, but it accounts for the majority of severe vision loss in AMD. The clinical features include:

SUDDEN ONSET

Rapid vision loss: The patient may experience a sudden and severe loss of their central vision.

Distortion: Straight lines may appear wavy or distorted. This is a symptom that is known as metamorphopsia. This is often one of the earliest signs of wet AMD.

SYMPTOMS

Choroidal neovascularisation: New, abnormal blood vessels grow from the choroid (a layer of blood vessels beneath the retina) into the subretinal space. These vessels are fragile, and they are prone to leaking fluid and blood.

Subretinal haemorrhage and fluid accumulation: There is leakage from these abnormal vessels causing the fluid and blood to accumulate under the retina, leading to swelling and damage.

Localised elevation: Parts of the macula may appear elevated as a result of the accumulation of fluid and blood, visible during an eye examination.

ADVANCED STAGES

Disciform scarring: Untreated neovascularisation results in the formation of scar tissue under the macula, known as a disciform scar. This scarring causes permanent central vision loss.

Severe central vision loss: Patients may experience a significant and often irreversible loss of central vision, although peripheral vision is usually preserved.

GENERAL SYMPTOMS OF AGE-RELATED MACULAR DEGENERATION

Regardless of the type, there are common symptoms of AMD and these include:

- Blurred central vision, resulting in difficulty reading, recognising faces and performing activities that require sharp vision.

- Visual distortions, whereby objects may appear warped or distorted.

- Dark or empty areas, resulting in blind spots in the centre of vision.

- Difficulty adapting to low light, making it challenging to adjust from bright to dim lighting conditions.

Early detection and management are crucial to slowing the progression of the disease and maintaining quality of life. Regular eye examinations are important, especially for those who are at higher risk, to identify AMD in its early stages when treatment is most effective. While dry AMD progresses slowly and leads to gradual vision loss, wet AMD can cause rapid and severe central vision loss, making timely intervention essential.

Table 6.2 provides a table summarising the different clinical presentations of dry AMD and wet AMD. The table highlights the key differences in the clinical presentations of dry and wet AMD, helping to differentiate between the two forms of the disease based on their symptoms and progression.

Table 6.2 A summary of the differences between dry and wet age-related macular degeneration (AMD)

Feature	Dry (atrophic) AMD	Wet (neovascular/exudative) AMD
Prevalence	About 85–90% of AMD cases	About 10–15% of AMD cases
Onset and progression	Slow and gradual	Rapid and sudden
Early signs	Drusen (yellow deposits under the retina)	Distortion of straight lines (metamorphopsia)
Vision changes	Mild blurring, difficulty reading or recognising faces	Sudden and severe central vision loss
Pigment changes	Dark or light spots in vision	Not typically present
Drusen	Small yellow deposits increase in size and number	Usually not present
Geographic atrophy	Present in advanced stages	Not present
Central vision loss	Gradual loss of central vision	Severe and often rapid loss of central vision

Feature	Dry (atrophic) AMD	Wet (neovascular/exudative) AMD
Peripheral vision	Generally preserved	Generally preserved
Choroidal neovascularisation	Absent	Present. Abnormal blood vessels grow under the retina
Fluid and haemorrhage	Absent	Fluid and blood leakage under the retina
Localised elevation	Absent	Parts of the macula may appear elevated
Disciform scarring	Absent	Present in untreated cases, leading to permanent damage
Common symptoms	Difficulty reading, dark spots, trouble adjusting to low light	Rapid central vision loss, visual distortions
Visual distortions	Less common	Common (wavy or distorted lines)
Blind spots (scotomas) and visual distortions	Central blind spots in advanced stages	Central blind spots, more sudden in onset

Source: Adapted from Davey (2024); Royal National Institute of Blind People (2023b).

CLINICAL INVESTIGATIONS AND DIAGNOSIS

Diagnosing AMD involves a combination of patient history, visual assessments and advanced imaging techniques. The goal is to detect characteristic changes in the retina and to distinguish between the two forms of AMD.

HISTORY TAKING

Conducting a thorough patient history and symptom evaluation involves a systematic approach to gathering relevant information that can aid in diagnosing AMD (Peate 2019). The information gathered at this stage is subjective information; objective information will require ocular testing. This process typically takes place during an initial consultation with an ophthalmologist or optometrist.

INITIAL CONSULTATION

MEDICAL AND OCULAR HISTORY

- Age assessment: Determine the patient's age to assess their risk, as AMD primarily affects those over 50 years.

- Family history: Ask if any close relatives (parents, siblings) have been diagnosed with AMD or other retinal diseases. This helps identify genetic predispositions. Specific gene variations are known to be associated with higher AMD risk.

- Smoking history: Inquire about the patient's smoking habits, including current and past smoking. Quantify the duration and intensity of smoking to gauge the associated risk. Smokers are significantly more likely to develop AMD compared to non-smokers.

- Cardiovascular history: Collect information on any cardiovascular conditions such as hypertension, heart disease or high cholesterol. These conditions can contribute to AMD. Cardiovascular diseases can increase the risk of AMD. These diseases affect the blood vessels, including those supplying the retina.

- Diet and lifestyle: Discuss dietary habits, focusing on the intake of leafy greens, fish and other foods rich in antioxidants and omega-3 fatty acids. Assess lifestyle factors such as physical activity and exposure to sunlight. Patients should be asked about their exposure to sunlight and use of protective measures such use of sunglasses.

- Ocular history: Review any past eye conditions, surgery or trauma. Note any previous diagnoses of retinal diseases or other significant ocular issues.

- Medication review: Document all medications the patient is currently taking, including over-the-counter drugs and supplements. Certain medications can impact retinal health, such as corticosteroids. These can influence the progression of AMD. Obtaining a complete list of medications is essential.

SYMPTOM INQUIRY

- Blurred vision: Ask if the patient experiences any blurriness, particularly in the central vision. Determine if it affects one or both eyes.

- Visual distortions (metamorphopsia): An Amsler grid test is used where the patient looks at a grid of straight lines to check for wavy or distorted lines, indicating potential wet AMD (see Chapter 2 of this book and Needham 2019).

- Difficulty reading: Question the patient about their ability to read small print or books and whether they need more light than usual.

- Recognising faces: Determine if the patient has trouble recognising familiar faces, a common issue with central vision loss.

- Dark or empty areas (scotomas): Ask if the patient notices any dark or empty spots in their vision.

- Recent vision changes: Inquire about any sudden changes in vision, which might indicate wet AMD, versus gradual changes more typical of dry AMD.

- Adapting to low light: Assess if the patient has difficulty adjusting from bright to dim environments, which can indicate photoreceptor dysfunction.

STRUCTURED INTERVIEWS AND QUESTIONNAIRES

- Standardised questionnaires: Use structured questionnaires specifically designed to identify AMD symptoms and risk factors. These tools ensure a comprehensive evaluation and standardise the data collection process.

- Visual functioning index: Incorporate tools such as the Visual Functioning Questionnaire (VFQ-25) to assess the impact of vision loss on the patient's quality of life and daily activities.

DOCUMENTATION AND FOLLOW-UP

Record findings: Meticulously document all findings from the patient history, symptom inquiry and objective tests. A comprehensive patient profile is then created that will include risk factors, symptom severity and any detected retinal changes.

Patient education: Inform the patient about their condition, potential risk factors and the importance of regular monitoring and follow-up appointments.

Management plan: Develop a personalised management plan that places the patient at the centre, based on the findings. This may include lifestyle modifications, dietary recommendations, smoking cessation support and regular follow-up visits for monitoring disease progression.

Following this structured approach, those who offer care and support to people with AMD can effectively diagnose, differentiate between its forms and initiate appropriate management strategies to preserve the patient's vision and quality of life.

A meticulous patient history and symptom evaluation are essential in diagnosing AMD. This process not only aids in identifying risk factors and early symptoms but also guides the selection of appropriate diagnostic tests and management strategies. Early and accurate diagnosis can significantly improve patient outcomes through timely intervention and tailored treatment plans. Regular follow-ups and patient education on modifiable risk factors, such as smoking cessation and nutritional improvements, are critical components of AMD management.

EXAMINATION AND INVESTIGATIONS

Before any examinations are performed or the initiation of investigations, it is crucial to adhere to local policies and procedures regarding infection prevention and control, the provision of a chaperone and obtaining consent. Ensure compliance with protocols before examinations and investigations.

Infection Prevention and Control Adherence to guidelines: Before performing any examination or initiating investigations, those who offer care and support to people must follow local infection prevention and control guidelines. This includes hand hygiene, using personal protective equipment and ensuring that all instruments and surfaces are properly sanitised.
Minimising cross-contamination: Procedures should be in place to minimise the risk of cross-contamination between patients. This includes the use of disposable instruments when possible and the thorough sterilisation of reusable equipment.

Provision of a Chaperone Patient comfort and safety: A chaperone should be offered during examinations and investigations to ensure patient comfort and safety.
Policy adherence: The use of a chaperone should be in accordance with local policies, which outline the circumstances under which a chaperone is required and the responsibilities of the chaperone.
Documentation: The presence of a chaperone, including their name and role, should be documented in the patient's medical record. If a patient declines the offer of a chaperone, this should also be noted.

Obtaining Consent Informed consent: Prior to any examination or investigation, informed consent must be obtained from the patient. This involves explaining the procedure, its purpose, potential risks and benefits and addressing any questions or concerns the patient may have.

Documenting consent: Consent should be documented in the patient's medical record. For more invasive procedures, written consent may be required, in addition to verbal consent.

Respecting patient autonomy: Patients have the right to refuse any procedure or investigation. Their decision should be respected, and alternative options should be discussed if applicable.

Guidelines exist regarding the examination and investigations that may be used when making a diagnosis of AMD (Royal College of Ophthalmologists 2024; NICE 2018). The following investigations may be undertaken (see also Chapter 2 of this book):

VISUAL ACUITY TEST

- Purpose: Measures the clarity of vision.

- Method: Patients read letters on a Snellen chart to determine their ability to see at various distances.

- Significance: Helps in assessing the degree of central vision loss.

AMSLER GRID TEST

- Purpose: Detects visual distortions and central scotomas.

- Method: Patients view a grid of straight lines and report any areas where lines appear wavy, blurred or missing.

- Significance: Useful for detecting early signs of wet AMD.

FUNDOSCOPIC EXAMINATION (OPHTHALMOSCOPY)

- Purpose: Direct visualisation of the retina.

- Method: An ophthalmoscope or a slit lamp with a special lens is used to examine the retina.

- Findings: Identifies drusen, pigmentary changes, geographic atrophy (dry AMD) and signs of neovascularisation or haemorrhage (wet AMD).

OPTICAL COHERENCE TOMOGRAPHY

- Purpose: Provides high-resolution, cross-sectional images of the retina (Sanderson 2019).

- Method: Uses light waves to take detailed images of the retina's layers.

- Findings: Detects the presence of drusen, subretinal fluid, retinal thickening and geographic atrophy. In wet AMD, it identifies fluid leakage, retinal detachment and neovascular membranes.

FLUORESCEIN ANGIOGRAPHY

- Purpose: Highlights blood vessels in the retina and identifies abnormal blood vessel growth.

- Method: A fluorescent dye is injected into a vein and a special camera takes pictures of the retina as the dye circulates.

- Findings: Identifies areas of leakage from neovascular membranes, helping to diagnose wet AMD.

INDOCYANINE GREEN ANGIOGRAPHY

- Purpose: Provides additional imaging of the choroidal blood vessels.

- Method: Similar to fluorescein angiography, but uses indocyanine green dye, which is better for visualising deeper choroidal vessels.

- Findings: Useful in detecting choroidal neovascularisation, especially when fluorescein angiography is inconclusive.

FUNDUS AUTOFLUORESCENCE

- Purpose: Detects lipofuscin accumulation in the RPE.

- Method: Uses specific wavelengths of light to capture images of the retina's autofluorescent properties.

- Findings: Highlights areas of RPE damage and drusen, useful in assessing the progression of dry AMD.

ELECTRORETINOGRAPHY

- Purpose: Assesses the function of the retina.

- Method: Measures the electrical responses of the retina to light stimulation.

- Findings: Provides information on retinal health, although not commonly used for routine AMD diagnosis.

A comprehensive approach combining patient history, visual function tests and advanced imaging techniques is essential for diagnosing AMD. These investigations help differentiate between dry and wet AMD, assess the severity of the disease and guide appropriate treatment decisions. Early detection through regular eye examinations, especially for those at higher risk, can significantly improve outcomes by allowing timely intervention.

MANAGEMENT

The management of AMD requires a comprehensive approach that varies depending on the type and severity of the condition. The primary goals are to slow disease progression, manage symptoms and maintain the patient's quality of life.

DRY AGE-RELATED MACULAR DEGENERATION (ATROPHIC)

For patients with dry AMD, lifestyle and dietary modifications are important. Encouraging patients to stop smoking is crucial, as smoking significantly increases the risk of disease progression. A diet rich in leafy green vegetables, fish and foods high in antioxidants and omega-3 fatty acids may be beneficial (NICE 2018).

Regular monitoring is vital for managing dry AMD. Patients should be offered follow-up visits to monitor disease progression, including comprehensive eye examinations and visual acuity tests. Using an Amsler grid at home helps patients detect any changes in vision promptly. For those with advanced dry AMD, low vision aids such as magnifiers and high-contrast reading materials can help cope with vision loss and vision rehabilitation services can assist patients in adapting to changes and maintaining independence.

WET AGE-RELATED MACULAR DEGENERATION (EXUDATIVE OR NEOVASCULAR)

The primary treatment for wet AMD is anti-vascular endothelial growth factor (VEGF) therapy, involving intravitreal injections of agents, for example, ranibizumab, aflibercept or bevacizumab. These medications inhibit the growth of abnormal blood vessels and reduce leakage, stabilising or improving vision. Initially, injections are given monthly until the condition stabilises, followed by less frequent injections based on disease activity. Regular follow-up with optical coherence tomography imaging and visual acuity tests is essential to monitor treatment response and disease progression.

In some cases, photodynamic therapy with verteporfin may be used in conjunction with anti-VEGF therapy. This procedure involves using a photosensitising drug that is activated by laser light to target and destroy abnormal blood vessels.

Addressing complications is also important in caring for and managing those people with wet AMD. Anti-VEGF injections help manage macular oedema, but in cases where significant oedema persists, adjunctive treatments may be considered. In advanced cases where scar tissue forms under the macula, the focus moves to managing symptoms and providing supportive care.

GENERAL MANAGEMENT STRATEGIES

Patient education plays a significant role in the management of AMD. Informing patients about the disease, its progression and the importance of regular monitoring and adherence to treatment plans is essential. Advising patients on how to recognise symptoms of disease progression, such as sudden vision changes, and to seek prompt medical attention can make a significant difference in outcomes (Sanderson 2019; Needham 2019).

Supportive care is also important. Addressing the emotional and psychological impact of vision loss through counselling or support groups can be beneficial. Providing training in the use of adaptive strategies and devices helps patients maintain their independence and quality of life.

Offering people care and support with AMD requires a multifaceted approach that includes lifestyle modifications, regular monitoring, medical treatments and supportive care. Tailoring the management plan to the type and severity of AMD helps patients maintain their vision and quality of life while slowing disease progression. Early diagnosis and intervention are critical in achieving the best possible outcomes for patients with AMD.

HEALTH TEACHING

Health teaching for individuals with AMD is crucial to help them manage their condition effectively and maintain their quality of life. The provision of education should cover various aspects, from understanding the disease to practical strategies for coping with vision changes (see Table 6.3).

Effective health teaching for individuals with AMD involves a comprehensive approach that includes education about the disease, treatment options, self-monitoring, lifestyle adjustments and emotional support. By providing patients with the knowledge and tools they need, healthcare providers can help them manage their condition more effectively, maintain their quality of life and adapt to the challenges posed by AMD.

Table 6.3   Health teaching needs for people with age-related macular degeneration (AMD)

Health teaching need	Discussion
Understanding AMD	Disease explanation: Offer patients information about what AMD is, including its types and how it affects vision. Explain the role of the macula in central vision and how AMD leads to its deterioration.
	Disease progression: Describe how AMD progresses and what changes patients might experience in their vision. Help them understand the potential for disease progression and the importance of early detection.
Treatment and management	Treatment options: Provide detailed information on available treatments, such as anti-vascular endothelial growth factor injections, photodynamic therapy and dietary supplements. Explain how these treatments work, their benefits and potential side effects.
	Medication concordance: Emphasise the importance of following the prescribed treatment regimen, including attending regular appointments for injections or monitoring.
Monitoring and early detection	Self-monitoring: Teach patients how to use an Amsler grid to monitor for changes in their vision at home. Instruct them on what to look for, such as wavy or distorted lines and the importance of reporting any changes promptly.
	Regular check-ups: Stress the importance of regular eye examinations and follow-up visits to monitor the progression of AMD and adjust treatment as needed.
Lifestyle and dietary recommendations	Dietary modifications: Advise a diet rich in antioxidants, omega-3 fatty acids and vitamins that may help slow AMD progression. Recommend foods such as leafy greens, fish and nuts.
	Smoking cessation: Emphasise the significant impact of smoking on AMD and encourage patients to stop smoking. Provide resources and support for smoking cessation if needed.
Vision aids and rehabilitation	Low vision aids: Inform patients about various low vision aids, such as magnifiers, large-print books and electronic devices designed to assist with daily activities.
	Vision rehabilitation: Recommend vision rehabilitation services that can help patients adapt to vision loss, including training in the use of assistive technologies and strategies for maintaining independence.

(Continued)

Table 6.3   *(Continued)*

Health teaching need	Discussion
Emotional and psychological support	Emotional impact: Acknowledge the emotional and psychological impact of vision loss. Provide information about counselling services, support groups and resources to help patients cope with the changes in their vision.
	Community resources: Share information about community resources, organisations and support groups for individuals with AMD, which can offer additional support and social interaction.
Practical tips for daily living	Home modifications: Offer practical advice on modifying the home environment to enhance safety and ease of living, such as improving lighting, using high-contrast colours and organising frequently used items in accessible locations.
	Safety measures: Advise on safety measures to prevent falls and accidents, which are especially important due to vision changes.

Source: Adapted from Royal College of Ophthalmologists (2024), American Academy of Ophthalmology (2019) and NICE (2018).

CONCLUSION

Age-related macular degeneration represents a significant challenge in ocular health, affecting millions worldwide and leading to profound changes in vision, particularly among the elderly. Understanding AMD – its types, pathophysiology, risk factors and management strategies – is key for effective patient care and intervention.

Dry AMD or atrophic progresses slowly, characterised by drusen formation and RPE changes, leading to gradual vision loss. Wet AMD or exudative AMD presents with more acute vision changes due to choroidal neovascularisation and subsequent leakage and scarring. Despite the relative rarity of wet AMD compared to dry AMD, it accounts for the majority of severe vision loss, making early diagnosis and prompt treatment essential.

Management of AMD involves a multifaceted approach tailored to the type and severity of the disease. For dry AMD, lifestyle modifications such as smoking cessation, dietary adjustments and the use of specific supplements can slow progression and improve quality of life. Wet AMD requires more intensive treatment, including anti-VEGF therapy, photodynamic therapy and sometimes laser treatments to manage abnormal blood vessel growth and minimise vision loss.

Health teaching plays a vital role in managing AMD. Informing and supporting patients about the nature of the disease, available treatments and lifestyle changes is critical for effective disease management. Providing support through vision rehabilitation, low vision aids and psychosocial resources helps patients adapt to vision changes and maintain their independence.

Age-related macular degeneration is a complex condition with significant implications for vision and quality of life. Through early detection, individualised treatment plans and comprehensive patient education, this can help mitigate the effects of AMD, improve patient outcomes and enhance overall well-being.

GLOSSARY OF TERMS

Amsler grid: A tool used to monitor changes in vision, particularly helpful for detecting early signs of wet age-related macular degeneration.

Anti-vascular endothelial growth factor (VEGF) therapy: Treatment involving drugs that inhibit vascular endothelial growth factor (VEGF) to prevent abnormal blood vessel growth in wet age-related macular degeneration.

Choroidal neovascularisation: The formation of new blood vessels in the choroid layer beneath the retina, characteristic of wet age-related macular degeneration.

Disciform scar: A scar that forms under the macula in advanced cases of wet age-related macular degeneration due to chronic leakage and bleeding from abnormal blood vessels.

Drusen: Yellow deposits under the retina, common in dry age-related macular degeneration, that can interfere with the function of the retinal pigment epithelium.

Exudative age-related macular degeneration: Also known as wet age-related macular degeneration; characterised by the growth of abnormal blood vessels that leak fluid or blood under the retina.

Geographic atrophy: An advanced form of dry age-related macular degeneration where there is extensive loss of the retinal pigment epithelium and photoreceptors, leading to significant vision loss.

Low vision aids: Devices such as magnifiers and special glasses that help individuals with age-related macular degeneration maximise their remaining vision.

Macula: The central part of the retina responsible for detailed central vision.

Metamorphopsia: Visual distortion, often a symptom of wet age-related macular degeneration, where straight lines appear wavy or curved.

Neovascular age-related macular degeneration: Another term for wet age-related macular degeneration, highlighting the growth of new, abnormal blood vessels.

Optical coherence tomography: A non-invasive imaging test that uses light waves to take cross-sectional pictures of the retina, helping to diagnose and monitor age-related macular degeneration.

Photodynamic therapy: A treatment for wet age-related macular degeneration that involves using a photosensitising drug activated by laser light to destroy abnormal blood vessels.

Photoreceptors: Cells in the retina (rods and cones) that detect light and allow vision.

Pigment epithelium detachment: Elevation of the retinal pigment epithelium, which can occur in wet age-related macular degeneration.

Retinal pigment epithelium: A layer of cells that nourishes the retinal cells and is crucial for their health and function; damaged in age-related macular degeneration.

Scotoma: A blind spot in the visual field, often occurring in advanced age-related macular degeneration.

Visual acuity: A measure of the clarity or sharpness of vision, often tested to monitor the progression of age-related macular degeneration.

Wet age-related macular degeneration: A type of age-related macular degeneration characterised by the growth of abnormal blood vessels under the retina, leading to leakage, bleeding and rapid vision loss.

MULTIPLE CHOICE QUESTIONS

1. What is the most common early sign of age-related macular degeneration?
   a) Sudden vision loss
   b) Blurred or distorted central vision
   c) Loss of peripheral vision
   d) Night blindness

2. Which type of age-related macular degeneration is characterised by the growth of abnormal blood vessels?
   a) Dry age-related macular degeneration
   b) Wet age-related macular degeneration
   c) Geographic Atrophy
   d) Stargardt Disease

3. What are drusen?
   a) Fluid-filled sacs in the retina
   b) Scar tissue on the macula
   c) Yellow deposits under the retina
   d) New blood vessels growing in the eye

4. What does the Amsler grid help detect?
   a) Peripheral vision loss
   b) Retinal detachment
   c) Central vision distortion
   d) Somnambulism

5. What is photodynamic therapy with verteporfin used for?
   a) Treating dry age-related macular degeneration
   b) Treating wet age-related macular degeneration
   c) Correcting refractive errors
   d) Reducing intraocular pressure

6. What symptom is typically NOT associated with age-related macular degeneration?
   a) Metamorphopsia
   b) Scotoma
   c) Peripheral vision loss
   d) Central vision loss

7. In dry age-related macular degeneration, what accumulates between the retina and the choroid?
   a) Blood vessels
   b) Fluid
   c) Drusen
   d) Scar tissue

8. Which of the following is a major risk factor for age-related macular degeneration?
   a) Age over 60
   b) Childhood obesity
   c) High levels of physical activity
   d) Low-fat diet

9. **What is the role of the retinal pigment epithelium in the eye?**
   a) To provide nutrients to the photoreceptors
   b) To focus light onto the retina
   c) To produce tears
   d) To control the amount of light entering the eye

10. **Which lifestyle change can significantly reduce the risk of age-related macular degeneration progression?**
    a) Increasing sugar intake
    b) Stopping smoking
    c) Avoiding dairy products
    d) Reducing physical activity

REFERENCES

American Academy of Ophthalmology (2019). Age-related macular degeneration preferred practice pattern. https://www.aao.org/education/preferred-practice-pattern/age-related-macular-degeneration-ppp (accessed August 2024).

Davey, P. (2024). *Medicine at a Glance*, 5e. Oxford: Wiley

National Institute for Health and Care Excellence (2018). Age-related macular degeneration. https://www.nice.org.uk/guidance/ng82/resources/age related-macular-degeneration-pdf-1837691334853 (accessed August 2024).

Needham, Y. (2019). Ophthalmological disorders (Chapter 38). In: *Learning to Care* (ed. I. Peate). London: Elsevier.

Peate, I. (2019). *Fundamentals of Assessment and Care Planning for Nurses*. Oxford: Wiley.

Royal College of Ophthalmologists (2024). Commissioning guidance. Age related macular degeneration services: recommendations. https://www.rcophth. ac.uk/wp-content/uploads/2021/08/Commission ing-Guidance-AMD-Services-Recommendations. pdf (accessed August 2024).

Royal National Institute of Blind People (2023a). Best disease (Best vitelliform macular dystrophy). https:// view.officeapps.live.com/op/view.uk%2Fdocuments %2FBest_Disease_2023.docx&wdOrigin=BROWSEL INK (accessed August 2024).

Royal National Institute of Blind People (2023b). Understanding age related macular degeneration. https://view.officeapps.live.com/op/view.aspx? src=https%3A%2F%2Fmedia.rnib.org.uk% 2Fdocuments%2FUnderstanding_AMD_2023.do cx&wdOrigin=BROWSELINK (accessed August 2024).

Royal National Institute of Blind People (2024). Stargardt disease. https://view.officeapps.live. com/op/view.aspx?src=https%3A%2F%2Fmedia. rnib.org.uk%2Fdocuments%2FStargardt_ Disease_2024.docx&wdOrigin=BROWSELINK (accessed August 2024).

Sanderson, A. (2019). Nursing patients with disorders of the eye and sight impairment (Chapter 14). In: *Alexander's Nursing Practice*, 5e (ed. I. Peate). London: Elsevier.

Sanderson, A. (2021). Providing eye care (Chapter 27). In: *The Nursing Associate's Handbook of Clinical Skills* (ed. I. Peate). Oxford: Wiley.

RETINAL DYSTROPHIES

Retinal dystrophies are a group of inherited disorders that affect the retina, the light-sensitive layer that is located at the back of the eye. These disorders are characterised by progressive loss of vision due to the degeneration of retinal cells (Royal National Institute of Blind People 2022). Inherited retinal degenerations encompass a diverse group of diseases with varying genetic and phenotypic characteristics. These conditions are marked by a progressive loss of photoreceptor function, leading to gradual vision loss (American Academy of Ophthalmology 2022).

TYPES

RETINITIS PIGMENTOSA

Affects the rod photoreceptors first, leading to night blindness and peripheral vision loss, eventually affecting the cone photoreceptors and resulting in central vision loss. This is the most common of the inherited retinal dystrophies (Royal National Institute of Blind People 2022; Borooah and Tint 2023).

STARGARDT DISEASE

A form of macular degeneration that typically begins in childhood or adolescence, leading to progressive central vision loss.

LEBER CONGENITAL AMAUROSIS

Presents in infancy with severe vision impairment or blindness and is often associated with other systemic abnormalities.

CONE–ROD DYSTROPHY

Involves both the cone and rod photoreceptors, usually starting with central vision loss and followed by peripheral vision loss.

CHOROIDERAEMIA

Affects the choroid, retinal pigment epithelium and retina, leading to night blindness and progressive vision loss.

BEST DISEASE (VITELLIFORM MACULAR DYSTROPHY)

Leads to progressive central vision loss due to the build-up of yellow pigment in the macula.

SYMPTOMS

- Night blindness: Difficulty seeing in low light conditions.

- Peripheral vision loss: Tunnel vision, where the side vision diminishes.

- Central vision loss: Difficulty with seeing details directly in front of the field of vision.

- Colour vision deficiency: Problems distinguishing colours.

- Photophobia: Sensitivity to light.

CAUSES

Retinal dystrophies are primarily caused by genetic mutations that affect the function and health of retinal cells (see Figure 7.1; National Eye Institute 2023). This means that the genetic mutations causing retinal dystrophies can be passed down from parents to their children in three different ways:

1. Autosomal dominant

2. Autosomal recessive

3. X-linked manner

There are a range of tests that can be undertaken to help to make a diagnosis of retinitis. Currently, there is no cure for retinal dystrophies, but several approaches can help manage the condition. This chapter will focus on retinitis pigmentosa.

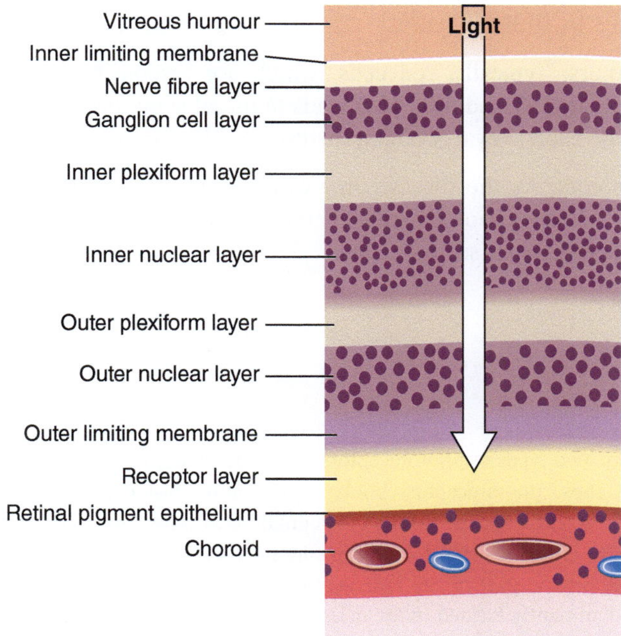

FIGURE 7.1   Retinal layers

PATHOPHYSIOLOGICAL CHANGES ASSOCIATED WITH RETINITIS PIGMENTOSA

The term retinitis pigmentosa comes from the distinctive characteristics of the disease observed during its early description.

- Retinitis: The suffix 'itis' typically indicates inflammation. Historically, many conditions affecting the retina were named with this suffix, even though retinitis pigmentosa is not an inflammatory disease. The prefix 'retina' refers to the part of the eye affected.

- Pigmentosa: This refers to the pigmentation or deposits of pigment that are seen in the retina. In retinitis pigmentosa, these pigment deposits are visible during an eye examination and they appear as dark, clumped pigments, particularly in the mid-peripheral retina. These pigment changes are due to the degeneration of the retinal pigment epithelium and the migration of pigment-laden cells into the retina.

Retinitis pigmentosa thus describes a condition that is characterised by retinal degeneration accompanied by distinctive pigmentary changes observed in the retina. Retinitis pigmentosa involves a series of pathological changes that occur in the retina, leading to progressive vision loss. These are the key pathophysiological changes that are associated with retinitis pigmentosa.

GENETIC MUTATIONS

- Underlying cause: Retinitis pigmentosa is caused by mutations in various genes essential for the normal function and survival of photoreceptors (rods and cones) and other retinal cells.

- Common genes: Mutations in genes such as *RHO*, *RPGR* and *USH2A* are frequently involved.

PHOTORECEPTOR DEGENERATION

- Rod photoreceptors: Typically, rod cells, which are responsible for night vision and peripheral vision, are affected first. This leads to initial symptoms of night blindness and loss of peripheral vision (Royal National Institute of Blind People 2017).

- Cone photoreceptors: As the disease progresses, cone cells, which are responsible for central vision and colour vision, also degenerate, leading to loss of central vision and difficulties in colour perception (see Box 7.1).

BOX 7.1	PHOTORECEPTORS

The retina contains two types of photoreceptors: rods and cones, named after their shapes. The outer segment of these photoreceptors holds light-sensitive visual pigment molecules called opsins, organised in stacked discs in rods and invaginations in cones. Vitamin A is crucial for these visual pigments. The retina has about 7 million cones and 120 million rods. Cones, concentrated in the macula (the central part of the retina), enable colour vision and the perception of fine details. Rods, predominantly located in the mid-peripheral and peripheral retina, are responsible for peripheral vision and seeing in low-light conditions, but they do not detect colours.

Source: Adapted from Meakin and Seewoodhary (2022).

RETINAL PIGMENT EPITHELIUM CHANGES

- Pigment migration: As photoreceptors degenerate, pigment-laden cells from the retinal pigment epithelium and retinal pigment epithelium migrate into the retina, forming characteristic clumps of pigment, often described as bone spicule-like deposits.

- Retinal pigment epithelium dysfunction: The retinal pigment epithelium, which supports photoreceptor function and health, becomes dysfunctional, exacerbating photoreceptor death.

VASCULAR CHANGES

- Attenuation of retinal blood vessels: Progressive narrowing of the retinal blood vessels is observed, which reflects the reduced metabolic demand due to photoreceptor loss.

- Reduced blood flow: As the photoreceptors and other retinal cells degenerate, the overall retinal blood flow decreases, contributing to further retinal atrophy.

RETINAL REMODELLING

- Glial cell activation: Müller cells and other glial cells in the retina become activated in response to photoreceptor death. These cells undergo hypertrophy and may contribute to the formation of scar tissue.

- Structural changes: The architecture of the retina becomes disrupted, with thinning of the outer retinal layers where photoreceptors reside and eventual involvement of inner retinal layers.

INFLAMMATORY RESPONSES

- Microglial activation: Microglial cells, the resident immune cells of the retina, become activated in response to photoreceptor death and debris. This activation can contribute to local inflammation and further photoreceptor damage.

SECONDARY EFFECTS

- Optic nerve atrophy: Prolonged degeneration of photoreceptors and other retinal cells can lead to atrophy of the optic nerve, which further impairs visual signal transmission to the brain.

CLINICAL IMPLICATIONS

The initial symptom of retinitis pigmentosa is typically night blindness, caused by the loss of rod photoreceptors. As the disease progresses and more rods degenerate, peripheral vision diminishes, leading to tunnel vision. In the later stages, cone photoreceptors are also affected, resulting in central vision loss. Additionally, as the cones deteriorate, there is a decline in visual acuity and colour vision, impacting the sharpness of vision and the ability to distinguish colours.

Understanding these pathophysiological changes is crucial for developing targeted therapies aimed at slowing down the progression of retinitis pigmentosa, preserving photoreceptor function and potentially restoring vision through interventions such as gene therapy, retinal implants or stem cell therapy.

EPIDEMIOLOGY

Retinitis pigmentosa is the most prevalent inherited retinal disease, affecting over 1.5 million people globally, though it is still classified as a rare disease. Prevalence rates for inherited retinal disease differ across Europe: in Spain, the rate is reported as less than 1 in 7000, while in Denmark and Norway, it is approximately 1 in 3000–4000. In the UK, retinitis pigmentosa affects an estimated 1 in 3000–4000 individuals. Globally, retinitis pigmentosa prevalence estimates range from 1 in 4000 to 1 in 3745. In the largest European countries, diagnosed patient estimates vary from 23 927 in Germany to 3617 in Spain, with non-syndromic retinitis pigmentosa representing 70–80% of all retinitis pigmentosa cases (Cross, van Steen, and Zegaoui 2022).

RISK FACTORS

Retinitis pigmentosa is a complex inherited retinal disorder that is influenced by several genetic and environmental factors. Having an understanding of these risk factors is crucial for early diagnosis, management and the provision of support services for those individuals affected as well as their families.

GENETIC MUTATIONS

FAMILY HISTORY

The most significant risk factor for retinitis pigmentosa is a family history of the disease or related inherited retinal conditions. If a parent, sibling or close relative has retinitis pigmentosa, the risk of developing the condition increases substantially. This strong familial link highlights the importance of genetic counselling for those with a known history of retinitis pigmentosa. Genetic counselling is a process where a person can obtain information and support about genetic conditions (Macmillan Cancer Support 2022). A genetic counsellor can help people understand their risk of developing or passing on, discuss genetic testing options and interpret test results.

INHERITED MUTATIONS

Retinitis pigmentosa can result from mutations in various genes, inherited in different patterns:

- Autosomal dominant: In this inheritance pattern, only one copy of the mutated gene from either parent is needed to cause the disorder. A child has a 50% chance of inheriting the condition if one parent is affected. Autosomal dominant retinitis pigmentosa often presents with a later onset and slower progression compared to other forms.

- Autosomal recessive: Two copies of the mutated gene, one from each parent, are necessary to cause the disorder. Typically, both parents are carriers of the gene but do not show symptoms themselves. There is a 25% chance their child will be affected. Autosomal recessive retinitis pigmentosa usually presents with an earlier onset and more rapid progression.

- X-linked: This form of inheritance occurs when the mutated gene is located on the X chromosome. Males (who have one X and one Y chromosome) are more likely to be affected, while females (who have two X chromosomes) are typically carriers and may or may not exhibit mild symptoms. A carrier mother has a 50% chance of passing the gene to her sons (who will be affected) and a 50% chance of passing it to her daughters (who will be carriers). X-linked retinitis pigmentosa tends to be more severe in males and often leads to early onset of symptoms; being male is therefore a risk factor.

GENETIC VARIABILITY

The specific gene and type of mutation can significantly impact the severity and progression of retinitis pigmentosa. Some mutations lead to a more aggressive form of the disease, resulting in a person experiencing more rapid vision loss, while in others it may cause a milder condition with slower progression. For example, mutations in the *RHO* gene often result in a more severe phenotype, whereas mutations in other genes, such as USH2A, might present with a slower progression.

PHENOTYPIC VARIABILITY

Even within the same family, individuals with the same genetic mutation can experience different symptoms and progression rates. This variability would suggest that other genetic modifiers, environmental factors and individual differences in gene expression may influence the disease's course. Researchers are actively studying these modifying factors to better predict disease progression and develop personalised treatment strategies.

ENVIRONMENTAL AND LIFESTYLE FACTORS

Although retinitis pigmentosa is primarily genetic, certain environmental and lifestyle factors can affect the overall health of the retina and therefore potentially influence the progression of the disease:

- Exposure to bright light. Chronic exposure to intense light may accelerate retinal damage in individuals with retinitis pigmentosa, although this remains a subject of research. Protecting the eyes from excessive light exposure by wearing sunglasses and avoiding prolonged exposure to bright light sources may be beneficial.

- A diet lacking essential nutrients, particularly those vital for retinal health (such as vitamin A), might impact the progression of retinal diseases, including retinitis pigmentosa. Ensuring an adequate intake of vitamin A and other antioxidants is important for retinal health. However, excessive vitamin A intake should be avoided unless prescribed due to potential harmful effects, especially since some forms of retinitis pigmentosa are not responsive to vitamin A supplementation and can even be worsened by it. The evidence regarding the use of nutritional supplements and their effectiveness is variable and generally limited (Sahni, Angi, and Irigoyen 2011).

- Factors that increase oxidative stress, such as smoking, may negatively impact retinal health and could potentially influence retinitis pigmentosa progression. Reducing oxidative stress through a healthy lifestyle, including a balanced diet rich in antioxidants, regular exercise and avoiding smoking, can support overall retinal health and it may help slow down disease progression.

AGE OF ONSET

EARLY ONSET

The earlier the person's symptoms appear, the more severe and rapid the progression of the disease tends to be. Early-onset retinitis pigmentosa often leads to significant vision loss during childhood or adolescence. This has the potential to affect the quality of life and educational and career opportunities.

LATE ONSET

Conversely, late-onset retinitis pigmentosa typically progresses more slowly, which allows individuals to retain functional vision for a longer period. This form of retinitis pigmentosa often presents during adulthood and can result in a gradual decline in vision over a number of years.

The primary risk factor for retinitis pigmentosa is genetic, with family history and specific gene mutations playing crucial roles in the condition. While environmental and lifestyle factors might influence the progression, the genetic component remains the most significant determinant in the development and course of retinitis pigmentosa. Understanding these risk factors can aid in early diagnosis, genetic counselling and the development of targeted therapies, ultimately improving the management and quality of life for individuals affected by retinitis pigmentosa.

CLINICAL PRESENTATION

Retinitis pigmentosa is a progressive retinal degenerative disorder that is characterised by a variety of symptoms that change over time. The clinical presentation can vary significantly depending on the specific type of retinitis pigmentosa, the age at which symptoms begin and the rate of disease progression.

INITIAL SYMPTOMS

NIGHT BLINDNESS

This is often one of the first symptoms that is noticed (Davey 2024). Patients may struggle to see in dimly lit environments, such as during dusk or at night. This difficulty is due to the degeneration of rod photoreceptors, which are essential for low-light vision. Rod cells, located mainly in the peripheral retina, are the first to be affected by the disease.

PERIPHERAL VISION LOSS

A gradual reduction in peripheral vision can manifest as a loss of the ability to detect objects or movement in the periphery of the person's visual field. The decline in peripheral vision results from the ongoing deterioration of rod photoreceptors. This loss is often first noticed by a patient as difficulty navigating in low-light conditions or a reduced ability to see objects outside the central field of vision.

PROGRESSIVE VISION LOSS

As retinitis pigmentosa advances, there is a loss of peripheral vision, which becomes more pronounced and leads to a 'tunnel vision' effect where the field of vision narrows to a central core (Galloway et al. 2023). As the progression of rod cell loss continues, this leads to a more constricted visual field. Patients may have difficulty in seeing anything outside a central area; this can impact their ability to detect objects or movement around them.

LOSS OF CENTRAL VISION

In the later stages of retinitis pigmentosa, patients may begin to experience a significant decline in their central vision, which affects their ability to see fine details directly in front of them. This occurs as cone photoreceptors, which are responsible for central and detailed vision, start to degenerate. The loss of cones affects tasks that require sharp vision, such as reading recognising faces or driving.

ADDITIONAL VISUAL SYMPTOMS

Colour Vision Deficiency   Patients with retinitis pigmentosa may experience difficulty distinguishing between colours, particularly as the disease progresses. The cone photoreceptors, which are crucial for colour vision, are progressively affected. This results in a decreased ability to perceive and differentiate colours accurately.

Reduced Visual Acuity   Visual acuity, or the sharpness of vision, tends to decline as retinitis pigmentosa progresses. Patients may find that it has become harder to see clearly even if they are using corrective lenses. The degeneration of both rod and cone cells leads to a general reduction in the clarity and detail of vision.

OTHER CLINICAL FEATURES

Photophobia   Some individuals with retinitis pigmentosa may develop an increased sensitivity to bright lights; this is known as photophobia (Royal National Institute of Blind People 2017). The changes that occur in retinal function and possibly along with the loss of certain photoreceptors can make bright lights uncomfortable or blinding.

Retinal Changes   Clinical examination of the retina might reveal specific changes that have occurred, such as 'bone spicule' pigmentation, where pigment accumulates in a pattern that resembles bone spicules (these resemble tiny, fragmented pieces of bone). There may also be thinning of the retinal layers and narrowing of retinal blood vessels. These changes reflect the ongoing loss and damage to retinal cells, primarily rod photoreceptors and can be visualised using specialised imaging techniques such as fundus photography or optical coherence tomography (Royal National Institute of the Blind 2017).

Electroretinogram Findings   The electroretinogram is a test that measures the electrical responses of the retina to light stimuli. In retinitis pigmentosa, electroretinogram results often show reduced or abnormal responses, indicating impaired retinal function. The decreased electrical activity that has been identified reflects the loss and dysfunction of photoreceptors, both rods and cones.

AGE OF ONSET AND PROGRESSION

Early-Onset Retinitis Pigmentosa   When retinitis pigmentosa symptoms appear during childhood or adolescence, the disease often progresses more rapidly, leading to significant vision loss earlier in life. Early-onset retinitis pigmentosa can affect educational and social development, requiring more intensive interventions and support.

Late-Onset Retinitis Pigmentosa If the symptoms develop in adulthood, the progression is generally slower; this can allow individuals to maintain useful vision for a longer period. Late-onset retinitis pigmentosa can impact daily life and activities gradually, with a more extended period of functional vision compared to early-onset cases.

In summary, the clinical presentation of retinitis pigmentosa involves a progressive decline in vision that typically starts with night blindness and peripheral vision that are due to the loss and degeneration of rod photoreceptors. As the disease advances, central vision and colour vision are affected. This is due to cone photoreceptor loss. Additional features may also be present such as photophobia; specific retinal changes and abnormal electroretinogram findings further characterise the disease. The age at which symptoms begin can significantly impact the severity and progression of vision loss, influencing the management and support strategies that are required. Understanding these clinical aspects can help in making a diagnosis, monitoring and developing appropriate interventions for those people with retinitis pigmentosa.

CLINICAL INVESTIGATIONS AND DIAGNOSIS

Diagnosing retinitis pigmentosa involves a series of clinical investigations to confirm the presence of the disease, make an assessment of its progression and to develop an understanding of its impact on the patient's vision. These investigations will often include a combination of patient history, visual function tests, retinal imaging and genetic testing (Royal National Institute of Blind People 2017).

PATIENT HISTORY

When diagnosing retinitis pigmentosa, it is important to undertake a comprehensive medical history, which is essential for identifying the disease, understanding its progression and differentiating it from other conditions. The medical history-taking component should address a range of topics that are related to symptoms, disease progression, family history and relevant past medical information.

SYMPTOM ONSET AND PROGRESSION

NIGHT BLINDNESS (NYCTALOPIA)

- One of the earliest symptoms in retinitis pigmentosa is difficulty seeing in low-light conditions or at night.

- History details: Ask when the patient had first noticed problems with night vision and how these difficulties have progressed. Night blindness in retinitis pigmentosa often starts early in the disease course.

- Questions to ask:

  - 'When did you first begin having trouble seeing in low light or at night?'

  - 'How has this difficulty changed over time? Has it worsened or has it remained stable?'

PERIPHERAL VISION LOSS

- Those patients with retinitis pigmentosa will often experience a progressive narrowing of the visual field. This is described as 'tunnel vision'.

- History details: Inquire about when the patient first noticed the issues with peripheral vision, such as bumping into objects or difficulties with side vision. This can help in gauging the extent of peripheral vision loss and tracking its progression.

- Questions to ask:
  - 'When did you first notice a reduction in your side vision?'
  - 'Have you had any issues with peripheral vision that have become more noticeable over time?'

CENTRAL VISION CHANGES

- In later stages, retinitis pigmentosa can affect central vision, impacting tasks that require detailed vision, such as reading or recognising faces.

- History details: Collect information about any changes in central vision, including any difficulties the patient may have with activities requiring sharp vision. Note the onset and the progression of these changes.

- Questions to ask:
  - 'Have you noticed any difficulties with reading or seeing fine details?'
  - 'When did you start having trouble with central vision and how has it changed?'

FAMILY HISTORY

GENETIC AND HEREDITARY PATTERNS

- Retinitis pigmentosa can be inherited in different patterns, such as autosomal dominant, autosomal recessive or X-linked. Obtaining a family history helps to identify the genetic basis of the disease.

- History details: Ask the patient about any relatives with similar vision problems or any family members who have been diagnosed with retinal conditions. This can help determine if the retinitis pigmentosa is part of a genetic syndrome or if it follows a particular inheritance pattern.

- Questions to ask:
  - 'Do any of your family members have retinitis pigmentosa or similar vision problems?'
  - 'Have any relatives been diagnosed with other genetic conditions that affect their vision?'

PREVIOUS OCULAR AND MEDICAL HISTORY

PRIOR EYE CONDITIONS

- Other eye conditions or previous ocular trauma might mimic or complicate retinitis pigmentosa.

- History details: Ask the patient about any past eye issues, any eye surgery or treatments that could impact the diagnosis or the management of retinitis pigmentosa.

- Questions to ask:
  - 'Have you had any previous eye conditions or surgery on the eye?'
  - 'Have you been treated for any other retinal or visual problems?'

SYSTEMIC HEALTH AND MEDICATIONS

- There are certain systemic conditions and medications that might impact retinal health or they may mimic retinitis pigmentosa symptoms.

- History details: Obtain information on systemic diseases the patient may have as well as a history of current medications, as these could influence the diagnosis or contribute to visual symptoms.

- Questions to ask:
  - 'Do you have any health conditions?'
  - 'Are you currently taking any medication or undergoing any treatment that might affect your vision?'

VISUAL FUNCTION IMPACT

DAILY LIFE AND FUNCTIONALITY

- Understanding how visual symptoms impact a person's daily life helps in assessing the severity of the condition and planning appropriate interventions.

- History details: Ask about how vision problems affect daily activities, employment and overall quality of life.

- Questions to ask:
  - 'How have your vision problems affected your daily activities and work?'
  - 'Are there specific tasks or activities that have become more challenging as a result of your vision changes?'

PSYCHOSOCIAL ASPECTS

EMOTIONAL AND PSYCHOLOGICAL IMPACT

- Chronic vision loss can have a significant emotional and psychological impact on the person, their family and carers.

- History details: Explore with the patient (and if appropriate family and carers) how the condition has affected their mental health, coping strategies and support systems.

- Questions to ask:

  - 'How are you?'

  - 'Do you think your vision loss has affected your emotional well-being and mental health?'

  - 'Do you have any support systems in place, such as family, friends or counselling?'

A thorough medical history is vital for diagnosing patients with retinitis pigmentosa. It involves documenting the onset and progression of symptoms such as night blindness, any peripheral vision loss and central vision changes. Gathering a detailed family history can help in identifying hereditary patterns and genetic factors. Evaluating previous ocular and medical history, understanding the impact the condition is having on daily life and addressing any psychosocial aspects are important when making a comprehensive assessment. This detailed history taking aids in accurate diagnosis, effective management and appropriate support for individuals with retinitis pigmentosa.

EXAMINATION AND INVESTIGATIONS

There are a number of examinations and investigations that can be used to make a diagnosis of retinitis pigmentosa. Specialist health and care providers as well as specialist equipment may be required. Local policy and procedure must be adhered to with regard to consent, infection prevention and control and the provision of a chaperone.

CLINICAL EXAMINATION

A visual acuity test measures the sharpness of vision in order to detect any decline in central vision. The visual field test is used to assess peripheral vision loss, which is often an early sign of retinitis pigmentosa. A colour vision test is undertaken to evaluate the ability to perceive colours, which can be affected in later stages of retinitis pigmentosa.

RETINAL IMAGING

FUNDUS PHOTOGRAPHY

- Provides a detailed image of the retina, allowing for the visualisation of characteristic retinitis pigmentosa changes such as bone spicules, retinal vessel attenuation and optic disc pallor.

- This helps in documenting the extent of retinal degeneration and tracking disease progression.

OPTICAL COHERENCE TOMOGRAPHY

- Optical coherence tomography uses light waves to create cross-sectional images of the retina, thereby revealing detailed structural information.

- Detects thinning of the retinal layers and loss of photoreceptors, which are indicative of retinitis pigmentosa.

FUNDUS AUTOFLUORESCENCE

- An imaging technique that shows the distribution of lipofuscin in the retinal pigment epithelium.

- Identifies those areas of retinal pigment epithelium damage and photoreceptor loss, providing insight into disease progression.

FUNCTIONAL TESTS

ELECTRORETINOGRAPHY

- Measures the electrical responses of the retina to light stimuli.

- An important test for diagnosing retinitis pigmentosa, electroretinography shows reduced or absent responses from rod and cone photoreceptors, thus confirming the presence of retinal dysfunction.

DARK ADAPTATION TEST

- This test is a valuable tool that is used to assess how quickly the eyes can adjust from bright to dim lighting.

- It detects early rod photoreceptor dysfunction, often before significant vision loss occurs.

GENETIC TESTING

GENETIC SCREENING

Genetic testing is crucial for enhancing diagnostic and prognostic accuracy. It informs patients and families about specific inheritance risks and guides treatment decisions (American Academy of Ophthalmology 2022). Analyses of DNA identifies mutations in genes known to be associated with retinitis pigmentosa. Genetic screening confirms the genetic basis of the disease and provides information on inheritance patterns.

WHOLE-EXOME SEQUENCING OR TARGETED GENE PANELS

- These are more comprehensive genetic tests that can identify mutations in multiple genes related to retinitis pigmentosa. Look at all the important parts of the patient's DNA.

- They are useful tests for diagnosing retinitis pigmentosa in cases where specific gene mutations are not identified through standard genetic testing. They aim to find genetic causes when the exact problem is not known.

- Family members should be examined and tested as necessary or desired to establish the hereditary pattern.

ADDITIONAL TESTS

OPTICAL COHERENCE TOMOGRAPHY ANGIOGRAPHY

- This is a non-invasive imaging technique that has the ability to visualise blood flow in the retina.

- This test helps in assessing retinal and choroidal vascular health, which can be affected in advanced stages of retinitis pigmentosa.

VISUAL FIELD TESTING (PERIMETRY)

- Perimetry measures the extent of peripheral vision and identifies areas of vision loss.

- Used to monitor the progression of peripheral vision loss over time, providing valuable information for disease management.

Diagnosing retinitis pigmentosa requires a comprehensive approach that includes patient history, clinical examination, retinal imaging, functional tests and genetic testing. These investigations help confirm the diagnosis, determine the extent of retinal damage, identify the genetic cause and guide management and counselling strategies. Early and accurate diagnosis is crucial for managing retinitis pigmentosa and providing patients with appropriate care and support.

MANAGEMENT

There is no way to reverse damage caused by retinitis pigmentosa (Kumar, Banik, and Ohia 2024). The Royal National Institute of Blind People (2022) notes that there is no cure for retinitis pigmentosa or treatment to prevent it from progressing. Issues that tend to be more common in people with retinitis pigmentosa, such as cataracts, can often be treated. Treatments are designed to address specific genetic causes of the disease and different stages of degeneration. Some treatments specifically target the genes or mutations responsible for the disease (American Academy of Ophthalmology 2022).

Retinitis pigmentosa is usually confined to the eye but may also be part of a syndrome with non-ocular features. There are at least 30 different associated syndromes that have been identified. Patients with Usher syndrome often experience hearing loss, which can be either profound or partial and may be present from birth or develop later. Usher syndrome accounts for about half of all combined deaf blindness cases.

Sahni, Angi, and Irigoyen (2011) note that the management of retinitis pigmentosa focuses on slowing the disease's progression, providing tools to help with low vision and offering psychological support to those affected. Tools to help with low vision are designed to assist individuals in performing daily activities and improving their quality of life despite reduced visual acuity. The Royal National Institute of Blind People (2023) discusses how people can make the most out of their sight, including a discussion on low vision assessment. Low vision aids are designed to help individuals perform daily tasks and improve their quality of life despite reduced visual acuity.

Magnifiers come in various forms. Handheld magnifiers are portable and useful for close-up tasks such as reading, while stand magnifiers are stationary and provide a larger, more stable viewing area for detailed work. Electronic magnifiers, which use a camera to display enlarged text and images on a screen, offer adjustable magnification levels.

Reading aids include large print books, which have bigger text for easier reading, and audiobooks for those who find print challenging. Text-to-speech software converts written text into spoken words, making reading accessible for many.

Assistive technology plays a significant role in managing low vision. Screen readers are software programs that read aloud the text displayed on a computer screen or mobile device, while screen magnification software enlarges text and images on screens.

Optical aids include bioptic telescopes, which are small telescopic lenses mounted on glasses to assist with distance vision, such as reading signs or watching TV. Prism glasses use prisms to improve visual alignment and depth perception.

Proper lighting can also make a big difference. Task lighting, which provides focused, bright light, is ideal for close work such as reading, while night lights offer low-intensity illumination to help with visibility in dark environments.

Low vision devices, for example, electronic reading devices and video magnifiers, are designed to magnify and enhance text or objects, making them easier to see. Electronic reading devices are handheld or wearable and offer high-contrast images, while video magnifiers have a camera and screen for magnifying printed materials.

Adaptive strategies can greatly aid in managing low vision. Orientation and mobility training helps individuals navigate and move around safely, often with the assistance of specialised instructors. Labelling systems, using braille or large print labels, assist in identifying household items or medications.

Personal support tools such as canes or guide dogs can assist with navigation and mobility, enhancing independence and safety.

These tools and strategies collectively help individuals with low vision maintain their independence and improve their daily functioning.

GENE THERAPY

Gene therapy is an advanced treatment approach designed to tackle genetic disorders such as retinitis pigmentosa. The primary goal of gene therapy is to address the specific genetic mutations responsible for the disease (American Academy of Ophthalmology 2022). This is achieved through two main methods: delivering functional copies of the affected gene or modifying the expression of the faulty gene.

By introducing a working version of a gene that is defective in retinitis pigmentosa, gene therapy aims to replace or supplement the faulty gene. Alternatively, it may alter how the faulty gene is expressed to reduce its harmful effects or enhance the function of remaining healthy genes. The overall purpose is to either correct the genetic defect or mitigate its impact, thereby improving the function of retinal cells (Mukamal 2021).

Gene therapy for retinitis pigmentosa is largely in the experimental phase. Researchers are conducting clinical trials to test various therapies and evaluate their effectiveness. Some of these experimental therapies have shown promise, with initial results indicating potential improvements in treatment outcomes.

Gene therapy seeks to directly address the genetic causes of retinitis pigmentosa. While the field is still developing and many therapies are undergoing testing, early results are hopeful and suggest that gene therapy may become a significant tool in managing and potentially treating retinitis pigmentosa in the future.

Voretigene neparvovec is a type of gene therapy that uses a specially modified virus (called an adeno-associated virus vector) to deliver a healthy copy of the *RPE65* gene directly into the retina. This treatment has been shown to improve vision in patients with Leber congenital amaurosis, which is a severe form of retinal disease caused by mutations in the *RPE65* gene.

In the UK, this therapy is approved for treating a specific condition known as biallelic RPE65 mutation-associated retinal dystrophy, which means the disease is caused by mutations in both copies of the *RPE65* gene (National Institute for Health and Care Excellence 2019). Voretigene neparvovec is notable because it is the first gene therapy specifically approved for eye diseases in the UK, marking a significant milestone in the treatment of genetic retinal disorders.

HEALTH TEACHING

For individuals with retinitis pigmentosa, their health teaching needs will focus on managing the condition, maximising remaining vision and improving the overall quality of life (see Table 7.1).

Addressing these areas, individuals with retinitis pigmentosa can better manage their condition, make the most of their remaining vision and maintain an improved quality of life.

Table 7.1   Health teaching needs for people with retinitis pigmentosa

Health teaching need	Discussion
Understanding the condition	Provide the patient with an overview of the condition. Offer information about what retinitis pigmentosa is, how it affects vision and its progression.
	Explain the hereditary nature (the genetic aspects) of retinitis pigmentosa and the implications for family planning and genetic counselling.
Vision management	Offer instruction on how to use devices such as magnifiers, specialised glasses and electronic aids to enhance vision.
	Teach strategies for daily living tasks, such as organising the home to improve navigation and using contrast to aid visibility.
Eye care	Emphasise the need for regular eye examinations and the importance of routine eye check-ups to monitor disease progression and manage complications.
	Offer advice on protecting eyes from bright light and UV exposure, which can exacerbate vision problems.
Mobility and orientation	Offer training on safe navigation and mobility techniques to help with spatial awareness and independent movement; this may be through an occupational therapist.
	Advise the patient on the use of mobility aids such as canes or guide dogs (Guide Dogs for the Blind Association 2022) and technology such as GPS apps designed for people with visual impairments.
Psychological support	Provide/suggest support for dealing with the emotional and psychological impact of vision loss, including counselling and support groups.
	Offer advice regarding driving and direct the patient to the Driver and Vehicle Licencing Agency (https://www.gov.uk/guidance/visual-disorders-assessing-fitness-to-drive).
	Connect individuals with resources for mental health support and adaptive skills training.
Community resources	Inform the patient about local and national organisations that offer resources, advocacy and support for people with visual impairments.
Safety and emergency planning	Suggest modifications to the home environment to reduce hazards and improve accessibility.
	Develop plans for navigating emergencies, including how to seek help and use emergency services effectively.

CONCLUSION

Retinitis pigmentosa is a complex and challenging retinal disorder characterised by progressive vision loss due to the degeneration of photoreceptor cells in the retina. This chapter has explored the management of the person with retinitis pigmentosa, emphasising the need for a multifaceted approach that includes understanding the disease, using available treatments and implementing strategies to enhance the quality of life.

A thorough grasp of retinitis pigmentosa's genetic basis, clinical manifestations and progression is essential. This knowledge allows for an accurate diagnosis and helps in anticipating the disease trajectory. Genetic counselling and family history play key roles in identifying at-risk individuals and guiding care decisions.

While there is currently no cure for retinitis pigmentosa, several treatment modalities are available to manage symptoms and slow progression. These include emerging gene therapies such as voretigene neparvovec and the use of low vision aids. Ongoing research and clinical trials offer hope for new and improved therapies that may further enhance patient outcomes.

Addressing the needs of individuals with retinitis pigmentosa extends beyond medical management. Health education plays a vital role in empowering patients to maximise their remaining vision and adapt to daily challenges. Providing access to assistive technologies, psychological support and community resources ensures that individuals with retinitis pigmentosa can lead fulfilling and independent lives despite their visual impairments.

GLOSSARY OF TERMS

Adeno-associated virus: A type of virus used as a vector in gene therapy to deliver genetic material into cells.

Bone spicules: Pigment clumping in the retina that resembles bone spicules, indicative of retinal degeneration in retinitis pigmentosa.

Dark adaptation test: A test that measures how quickly the eyes adjust to low light conditions, often used to assess retinal function.

Electroretinogram: A diagnostic test that measures the electrical response of the retina to light stimuli, used to evaluate retinal function.

Fundus photography: A technique to capture detailed images of the retina to document and monitor changes associated with retinitis pigmentosa.

Gene therapy: A treatment method that involves correcting or replacing defective genes responsible for genetic disorders.

Inheritance patterns: The ways in which genetic mutations are passed from parents to offspring, including autosomal dominant, autosomal recessive and X-linked patterns.

Macula: The central part of the retina responsible for sharp, detailed vision, which can be affected in later stages of retinitis pigmentosa.

Night blindness (nyctalopia): Difficulty seeing in low-light conditions, often an early symptom of retinitis pigmentosa.

Photoreceptors: Specialised cells in the retina (rods and cones) that detect light and are affected in retinitis pigmentosa.

Retinal degeneration: The progressive loss of retinal cells leading to vision impairment, characteristic of retinitis pigmentosa.

Subretinal injection: A method of delivering treatments or gene therapy directly into the space beneath the retina.

Tunnel vision: A loss of peripheral vision resulting in a narrowed field of view, common in retinitis pigmentosa as the disease progresses.

Usher syndrome: A genetic disorder that combines retinitis pigmentosa with hearing loss, which can also affect quality of life.

Visual acuity: The sharpness or clarity of vision, which can decline as retinitis pigmentosa progresses.

X-linked inheritance: A pattern of inheritance where the defective gene is located on the X chromosome, affecting mainly men and passed from carrier mothers.

MULTIPLE CHOICE QUESTIONS

1. What is retinitis pigmentosa?
   - **a)** A type of bacterial infection
   - **b)** A progressive retinal degeneration disorder
   - **c)** A corneal disorder
   - **d)** An inflammatory eye condition

2. Which cells are primarily affected in retinitis pigmentosa?
   - **a)** Cone cells
   - **b)** Rod cells
   - **c)** Ganglion cells
   - **d)** Retinal pigment epithelium cells

3. Which of the following is a common early symptom of retinitis pigmentosa?
   - **a)** Blurred vision
   - **b)** Night blindness
   - **c)** Double vision
   - **d)** Sudden loss of vision

4. What is the purpose of a dark adaptation test?
   - **a)** To measure colour vision
   - **b)** To assess the retina's response to light changes
   - **c)** To evaluate peripheral vision
   - **d)** To detect cataracts

5. What is the primary aim of gene therapy for retinitis pigmentosa?
   - **a)** To replace defective genes with functional ones
   - **b)** To strengthen retinal blood vessels
   - **c)** To treat secondary infections
   - **d)** To improve eye muscle function

6. Which of the following is NOT a common diagnostic test for retinitis pigmentosa?
   - **a)** Fundus photography
   - **b)** Electroretinogram
   - **c)** Visual acuity test
   - **d)** MRI of the brain

7. What is a key characteristic observed in the fundus of a patient with retinitis pigmentosa?
   a) Retinal haemorrhages
   b) Bone spicules
   c) Macular oedema
   d) Cataracts

8. What visual function is primarily lost early in the course of retinitis pigmentosa?
   a) Colour vision
   b) Central vision
   c) Night vision
   d) Peripheral vision

9. What does a visual field test measure in patients with retinitis pigmentosa?
   a) The ability to see fine details
   b) The range of peripheral vision
   c) The response of the retina to light
   d) The thickness of the retina

10. What is the primary goal of using low vision aids in retinitis pigmentosa?
    a) To restore lost vision
    b) To slow disease progression
    c) To maximise the use of remaining vision
    d) To prevent further retinal damage

REFERENCES

American Academy of Ophthalmology (2022). Clinical statement, guidelines on clinical assessment of patients with inherited retinal degenerations. https://www.aao.org/education/clinical-statement/guidelines-on-clinical-assessment-of-patients-with (accessed August 2024).

Borooah, S. and Tint, N.L. (2023). The visual system (Chapter 8). In: *Macleod's Clinical Examination*, 15e (eds. A.R. Dover, J.A. Innes, and K. Fairhurst). London: Elsevier.

Cross, N., van Steen, C., and Zegaoui, Y. (2022). Retinitis pigmentosa: burden of disease and current unmet needs. *Clinical Ophthalmology* 16: 1993–2010. doi: 10.2147/OPTH.S365486.

Davey, P. (2024). *Medicine at a Glance*, 5e. Oxford: Wiley.

Galloway, N.R., Amoaku, W.M.K., Galloway, P.H. et al. (2023). Common Eye Diseases and their Management. Springer Nature. doi: 10.1007/978-3-031-08450-8_23.

Guide Dogs for the Blind Association (2022). Living with retinitis pigmentosa. https://www.guidedogs.org.uk/getting-support/information-and-advice/eye-conditions/retinitis-pigmentosa/living-with-retinitis-pigmentosa/ (accessed August 2024).

Kumar, P., Banik, S.P., and Ohia, S.E, (2024). Current insights on the photoprotective mechanism of the macularcarotenoids, lutein and zeaxanthin: safety, efficacy and bio-delivery. *Journal of American Nutrition Association* 43 (6): 505–518. doi: 10.1080/27697061.2024.2319090.

Macmillan Cancer Support (2022). Genetic counselling. https://www.macmillan.org.uk/cancer-information-and-support/worried-about-cancer/causes-and-risk-factors/what-is-genetic-counselling (accessed August 2024).

Meakin, S. and Seewoodhary, M. (2022). The person with an ear or eye disorder (Chapter 33). In: *Nursing Practice*, 3e (eds. I. Peateand and A. Mitchell). Oxford: Wiley.

Mukamal, R. (2021). New treatments for retinitis pigmentosa. American Academy of Ophthalmology. https://www.aao.org/eye-health/tips-prevention/gene-therapy-new-retinitis-pigmentosa-lca-luxturna (accessed August 2024).

National Eye Institute (2023). Retinitis pigmentosa. https://www.nei.nih.gov/learn-about-eye-health/eye-conditions-and-diseases/retinitis-pigmentosa (accessed August 2024).

National Institute for Health and Care Excellence (2019). Voretigene neparvovec for treating inherited retinal dystrophies caused by RPE65 gene mutations. https://www.nice.org.uk/guidance/hst11 (accessed August 2024).

Royal National Institute of Blind People (2017). Understanding retinitis pigmentosa. https://www.rcophth.ac.uk/wp-content/uploads/2020/05/Understanding-Retinitis-Pigmentosa_2017.pdf (accessed August 2024).

Royal National Institute of Blind People (2022). Inherited retinal dystrophies including retinitis pigmentosa. https://media.rnib.org.uk/documents/Understanding_Inherited_retinal_dystrophies_PT_2022_i0scuYn.pdf (accessed August 2024).

Royal National Institute of Blind People (2023). Making the most of your sight. https://media.rnib.org.uk/documents/Starting_Out_-_Making_the_most_of_your_sight_2023.pdf (accessed August 2024).

Sahni, J.N., Angi, M., and Irigoyen, C. (2011). Therapeutic challenges to retinitis pigmentosa: from neuroprotection to gene therapy. *Current Genomics* 12 (4): 276–284. doi: 10.2174/138920211795860062.

 # Presbyopia

MYOPIA, HYPEROPIA AND PRESBYOPIA

In a person who has myopia (short-sightedness), the lens is unable to focus the image onto the retina and the focus of the image falls short (Figure 1.9, Chapter 1 of this book). With myopia, people can see objects close to them but those that are far away are blurred. Myopia is easily corrected by the use of corrective lenses, either in the form of glasses or contact lenses (Clare 2020).

In the person with hyperopia (long-sightedness), the image is focused onto a point behind the retina (Figure 1.10, Chapter 1 of this book); therefore, these people can see things at a distance but not near to them.

Presbyopia is the loss of the ability to focus on close objects as the person ages. The most common theory for this is the loss of elasticity in the lens, age-related deterioration in near vision (Borooah and Tint 2023). The loss of the ability to focus on nearby objects occurs in everyone, but at different rates and with different effects on vision. The onset of presbyopia is most commonly noticed at 40–50 years of age. Presbyopia can be corrected using convex lenses, usually known as reading glasses, although they are corrective for all tasks that require near vision (Needham 2019).

The word 'presbyopia' comes from Greek roots. It combines 'presbys', meaning 'old man' or 'elder' and 'opia', meaning 'sight' or 'vision'. Therefore, presbyopia essentially means 'vision of the old man', reflecting the age-related difficulty in seeing up close that commonly occurs as people get older.

EMMETROPIA

Emmetropia is the term used to describe a person's vision when absolutely no refractive error or defocus exists. It refers to an eye that has no visual defects. Images formed on an emmetropic eye are perfectly focused, clear and precise. Eyes with emmetropia do not require vision correction. When a person has emmetropia in both eyes, the person is described as having ideal vision. When an eye is emmetropic, light rays coming into the eye from a distance come into perfect focus on the retina.

REFRACTIVE ERROR

If a person is not emmetropic, then they have a refractive error. See Table 8.1 for examples of refractive errors.

PATHOPHYSIOLOGICAL CHANGES ASSOCIATED WITH PRESBYOPIA

Presbyopia is a common age-related condition where the eye gradually loses the ability to focus on nearby objects. Uncorrected refractive error is a readily treatable cause of visual impairment (Little et al. 2024). This usually becomes noticeable around the age of 40 years, and it continues to progress with age. The underlying pathophysiological changes primarily involve the lens and surrounding structures of the eye. This leads to a diminished ability to accommodate or adjust focus for near vision.

Table 8.1 Refractory disorders

Example of refractive error	Discussion
Near-sightedness	Near-sightedness, or myopia, is a condition in which near objects are seen clearly, but distant ones are blurred. Near-sightedness can be inherited and is often discovered during childhood. However, you can develop near-sightedness in early adulthood. People who develop myopia in early adulthood usually do not develop high amounts of near-sightedness.
Farsightedness	Farsightedness or hyperopia (also referred to as hypermetropia) usually causes distant objects to be seen clearly, but close objects to appear blurred. Farsightedness often runs in families. When someone has higher levels of farsightedness, their distant vision may become blurry in addition to their near vision. Many people mistake farsightedness for presbyopia, the refractive error that usually occurs in people over 40 years of age.
Astigmatism	Astigmatism usually occurs when the cornea has an irregular curvature. The cornea is curved more in one direction, causing blurry vision. Astigmatism can cause blurry vision at all distances, and it often occurs along with farsightedness or near-sightedness. Most people have very small amounts of astigmatism. Larger amounts of astigmatism cause distortion in addition to blurry vision. People with very high levels of astigmatism sometimes have a difficult time achieving 20/20 vision.
Presbyopia	Presbyopia is the normal ageing process of the lens of the eye. It is the loss of elasticity of the lens that occurs with ageing, causing difficulty focusing at close ranges. It is believed that, in addition to the loss of elasticity of the lens, the muscle that makes the lens change focus, called the ciliary body, also starts to lose effectiveness. Presbyopia usually becomes significant after the age of 40–45 years; however, people between 35 and 40 years may exhibit early signs depending on their visual state, work and lifestyle.

Source: Adapted from Cooper and Tkatchenko (2018), Wang et al. (2018), Castagno et al. (2014) and Torricelli et al. (2012).

One of the central factors in presbyopia is the reduction in the elasticity of the lens. In younger individuals, the lens is highly flexible and can easily change its shape to focus on objects that are at varying distances. However, as people age, the lens becomes stiffer and it is less capable of changing its shape (Huether and Rodway 2019), this means that the lens cannot thicken sufficiently to focus on close objects, which is essential for near vision.

Additionally, changes occur in the ciliary muscle, which is responsible for altering the lens shape during accommodation (Jarvis and Eckhardt 2024), (see Box 8.1). With ageing, the ciliary muscle's strength and functionality decline. It also becomes more prone to fatigue, which reduces its efficiency in helping the lens adjust to near vision. The lens capsule, a membrane that surrounds the lens, also becomes less flexible with age. This further hinders the ability of the lens to change its shape (Little et al. 2024).

BOX 8.1   ACCOMMODATION

Mechanism of accommodation

Accommodation involves a complex interplay between the eye's anatomical structures and their functional adjustments.

1. The eye's anatomy involved in accommodation

- **Lens**: A transparent, flexible structure located behind the iris. Its primary role is to focus light onto the retina.
- **Ciliary muscle**: A ring-shaped muscle surrounding the lens. It controls the shape of the lens through contraction and relaxation.
- **Suspensory ligaments (zonules)**: Thin fibres that connect the ciliary muscle to the lens. They help hold the lens in place and transmit the ciliary muscle's force to the lens.

2. Accommodation for distant objects

When focusing on something far away, such as a road sign in the distance:

- **Ciliary muscle relaxation**: The ciliary muscle relaxes, reducing the tension on the suspensory ligaments.
- **Lens flattening**: The reduction in tension causes the lens to become flatter and thinner. This decreases its optical power, which is suitable for focusing on distant objects.
- **Light focus**: The flatter lens helps focus light rays from distant objects onto the retina, creating a sharp image.

3. Accommodation for near objects

When the focus is moved to a close object, such as a book:

- **Ciliary muscle contraction**: The ciliary muscle contracts, which reduces the pull of the suspensory ligaments on the lens.
- **Lens rounding**: The decrease in tension allows the lens to become more spherical and thicker. This increases its optical power, necessary for focusing on near objects.
- **Increased refractive power**: The more rounded lens helps converge light rays from near objects onto the retina, providing a clear image.

The accommodation reflex

The process of accommodation is part of a broader visual reflex called the accommodation reflex, which also involves:

- **Pupillary constriction**: The pupils constrict to improve the depth of field and reduce the amount of light entering the eye, which enhances focus on near objects.
- **Convergence**: The eyes turn inward slightly to maintain binocular vision and focus on the near object.

Changes with age and presbyopia

As we age, the eye undergoes changes that affect accommodation:

- **Lens hardening**: The lens becomes stiffer and less flexible, reducing its ability to change shape.

- **Ciliary muscle weakening**: The ciliary muscle's efficiency diminishes over time, making it harder to contract and adjust the lens's shape.

- **Reduced accommodation power**: These changes decrease the eye's ability to focus on close objects, leading to the condition known as presbyopia.

Importance of accommodation

Accommodation is crucial for:

- **Visual clarity**: It allows for sharp focus across a range of distances, making it possible to see both near and far objects clearly.

- **Everyday tasks**: Effective accommodation is essential for activities such as reading, sewing or using a smartphone, which require frequent shifts in focus.

Summary

The process of accommodation is a sophisticated mechanism involving the lens, ciliary muscle and suspensory ligaments to adjust focus between near and distant objects. Its effectiveness is vital for clear vision at varying distances and becomes a key consideration in addressing age-related changes such as presbyopia. Understanding how accommodation works helps in appreciating the challenges associated with ageing and in choosing appropriate corrective measures to maintain visual clarity.

Source: Adapted from Huether and Rodway (2019); Galloway et al. (2023).

The lens itself continues to grow throughout life; it does this by adding new layers, which leads to an increase in its thickness. This growth makes it more difficult for the ciliary muscles to induce the necessary changes in lens shape that are required for focusing on close objects. Consequently, the range over which the eye can accommodate decreases, leading to difficulties in near vision.

There are other age-related changes that can exacerbate presbyopia. The pupil, for instance, tends to become smaller with age, reducing the amount of light entering the eye, which impacts near vision, especially in low-light conditions. Changes in the vitreous body, which helps maintain the eye's shape, can also influence overall eye function and contribute to presbyopia.

The combination of these changes results in a progressive stiffening and thickening of the lens, along with a reduced functionality of the ciliary muscles and lens capsule. Together, these factors will lead to the diminished ability to focus on near objects, which is the hallmark of presbyopia.

Understanding the pathophysiology that is associated with presbyopia is crucial for developing effective management strategies and also for advancing research into potential treatments to mitigate or reverse this age-related condition.

EPIDEMIOLOGY

In 2019, there were at least 2.2 billion people around the world with a vision impairment, of whom at least one billion have a vision impairment that could have been prevented or is yet to be addressed (World Health Organization 2019). Refractive errors are the most common visual problem (Hagler et al. 2023). Presbyopia affects a substantial portion of the population and understanding its epidemiology is important for addressing vision impairment.

The Royal National Institute of Blind People (2021) offers statistics on visual impairment in the UK, including conditions such as presbyopia. There are more than two million people in the UK who are estimated to be living with sight loss. This level of sight loss is severe enough to significantly impact their daily lives, including difficulties in seeing objects at a distance and potentially needing to surrender their driving licenses. The more than two million people living with sight loss include:

- Individuals who are registered as blind or partially sighted.

- Those whose vision is better than the levels qualifying for registration.

- Individuals awaiting or undergoing treatment such as eye injections, laser treatment or surgery that may improve their sight.

- People whose sight loss could be improved by wearing correctly prescribed glasses or contact lenses.

Every day, 250 people in the UK begin to lose their sight. This equates to one person every six minutes. This statistic includes sight loss resulting from age-related macular degeneration, glaucoma and diabetic retinopathy, along with other causes of permanent and irreversible sight loss. Many more people will experience sight loss due to uncorrected refractive errors and cataracts, which includes those with presbyopia.

One in five people will live with sight loss at some point in their lifetime, assuming that the underlying risk factors associated with sight loss remain unchanged. Additionally, many more will experience sight loss due to eye injury, cataracts or refractive errors, which includes presbyopia.

The number of people with sight loss is projected to increase significantly. By 2050, it is predicted that sight loss will double to over four million. This projection assumes that the underlying risk factors associated with sight loss will remain unchanged and that broad demographic trends, such as an ageing population, will continue.

The main causes of sight loss among the more than two million people affected are:

- 23% (488 000 people) with age-related macular degeneration

- 19% (394 000 people) with cataracts

- 5% (97 000 people) with diabetic retinopathy

- 7% (151 000 people) with glaucoma

- 39% (809 000 people) with uncorrected refractive error

- 7% (155 000 people) with other eye problems

Understanding the epidemiology of presbyopia is important for effective public health planning, resource allocation, economic impact assessment, treatment improvement, policy-making, enhancing quality of life and future healthcare planning. This comprehensive understanding ensures that strategies and interventions are in place to manage and mitigate the impact of presbyopia on individuals and society.

RISK FACTORS

Presbyopia, an age-related decline in the eye's ability to focus on near objects, affects nearly everyone as they grow older. Although age is the primary risk factor for presbyopia, there are a range of other factors that can influence its onset and severity. Understanding these risk factors is important for the early identification and effective management of the condition.

AGE

The most significant risk factor for presbyopia is age. Typically, symptoms begin to appear in the early to mid-40s and progress over time. As the lens of the eye naturally loses its elasticity with age, it becomes harder to focus on close objects.

GENETICS

Genetic predisposition plays a role in the onset of presbyopia. Individuals with a family history of the condition may develop it earlier or experience it more severely. Genetics can affect the elasticity of the lens and the function of the ciliary muscles, contributing to presbyopia.

OCCUPATION

People who engage in extensive near-vision tasks, such as reading, writing or detailed arts and crafts, may experience presbyopia symptoms more acutely. Continuous close-up work can strain the eyes and this can potentially exacerbate symptoms, making them more noticeable.

REFRACTIVE ERRORS

Individuals with hyperopia (farsightedness) are more likely to experience presbyopia earlier than those with normal vision. Hyperopia places additional strain on the eyes when focusing on near objects, compounding the effects of presbyopia. Conversely, those with myopia (near-sightedness) might not notice presbyopia as early because they can see close objects clearly without correction. However, they will still develop presbyopia and may need separate correction for near vision as they age.

HEALTH CONDITIONS

Certain health conditions can accelerate the onset of presbyopia. Diabetes can affect the eye's lens and its ability to focus, leading to earlier onset. Cardiovascular diseases, which impact blood circulation, can also contribute to the condition. Neurological conditions, for example, multiple sclerosis, which affect the muscles and nerves involved in eye function, can similarly lead to early onset of presbyopia.

MEDICATIONS

Some medications can impact the eye's focusing ability, potentially accelerating presbyopia. Antidepressants and antihistamines can cause dry eyes or affect accommodation. Diuretics, used to treat high blood pressure and other conditions, can lead to changes in the eye's refractive status.

ENVIRONMENTAL FACTORS

Environmental factors, such as poor lighting conditions, can strain the eyes and make the symptoms of presbyopia more noticeable. Prolonged exposure to ultraviolet light can damage the eyes over time, accelerating the ageing process of the lens and contributing to presbyopia.

LIFESTYLE ACTORS

Certain lifestyle choices can influence the onset and progression of presbyopia. Smoking has been linked to a variety of eye conditions, including cataracts, which can compound the effects of presbyopia. Excessive alcohol consumption can lead to nutritional deficiencies that may affect eye health and potentially exacerbate the condition.

EYE SURGERY

Previous eye surgery can influence how presbyopia develops. Individuals who have undergone procedures such as laser-assisted in situ keratomileusis (LASIK), a type of refractive eye surgery, or cataract surgery may experience changes in their vision. While LASIK corrects distance vision, it does not prevent the natural ageing process of the lens.

GENDER

Women might experience presbyopia slightly earlier than men, possibly due to hormonal changes, particularly those associated with menopause. However, more research is needed to confirm this gender difference conclusively.

Presbyopia is an inevitable part of ageing, but its onset and severity can be influenced by various factors, including genetics, occupation, existing refractive errors, health conditions, medications, environmental factors, lifestyle choices, previous eye surgery and potentially gender. By understanding these risk factors, individuals can take proactive steps to manage and mitigate the impact of presbyopia. Regular eye examinations and healthy lifestyle choices are essential components of managing the risk and progression of presbyopia, ensuring better eye health and quality of life as people age.

CLINICAL PRESENTATION

The person may start to notice presbyopia shortly after the age of 40 years and often they will hold reading materials farther away in order to see them clearly.

Symptoms of presbyopia often impact daily activities, including difficulty with driving, reading (especially small print, such as medication instructions) and preparing meals. The progression of symptoms can be so gradual that individuals might not immediately notice changes in their vision. Instead, they may experience headaches or have red, sore or watery eyes. Table 8.2 presents the signs and symptoms of presbyopia.

Understanding the clinical presentation of presbyopia is vital for accurate diagnosis, effective management, improving patient quality of life, patient education, monitoring progress, advancing treatments and public health planning. It ensures that individuals receive timely and appropriate care, enhancing their overall visual health and well-being.

CLINICAL INVESTIGATIONS AND DIAGNOSIS

To diagnose presbyopia, a comprehensive clinical evaluation is necessary. This evaluation usually involves several key investigations and tests to assess visual function and rule out other potential causes of visual impairment.

Table 8.2   The signs and symptoms associated with presbyopia

Signs	Symptoms
Reduced near-vision acuity:	Difficulty reading small print:
Clinical examination with a near-vision chart will reveal reduced acuity at normal reading distances, typically starting at about 40 cm.	Individuals often notice difficulty reading small print, such as books, newspapers or labels on products. They may find themselves holding reading materials farther away to see them clearly.
Pupil constriction and accommodation tests:	Eyestrain:
Testing for the eye's ability to accommodate (change focus from far to near) will show reduced amplitude of accommodation. This is measured using techniques such as the push-up test or minus lens test.	Prolonged close-up activities, such as reading, sewing or working on a computer, can lead to eyestrain or fatigue. Symptoms may include headaches, burning or aching eyes, blurred vision and a feeling of tiredness.
Reading glasses or bifocals use:	Blurred vision at normal reading distance:
Patients may already be using over-the-counter reading glasses or bifocals as a compensatory measure for their symptoms.	Objects that are close, such as a smartphone screen or a menu, may appear blurry. This blurriness is typically worse in low-light conditions or after prolonged close work.
	Need for brighter lighting:
	Individuals with presbyopia may find that they need brighter lighting for reading or other close-up tasks. This is because increased light helps to improve contrast and clarity.
	Delayed focus change:
	There may be a noticeable delay in the ability to shift focus from distant to near objects. For example, looking at a computer screen after looking at something across the room may cause a brief period of blurriness.
	Frequent changes in prescriptions:
	People with presbyopia often experience frequent changes in their eyeglass or contact lens prescriptions as the condition progresses.

Source: Adapted from Cochrane, du Toit, and Le Mesurier (2010), Galloway et al. (2023) and Hagler et al. (2023).

PATIENT HISTORY

- Symptom inquiry: Detailed questioning about symptoms, including difficulties with near vision, reading small print and any associated discomfort such as headaches or eye strain.

- Lifestyle and visual habits: Information about daily activities, visual tasks and any recent changes in vision.

VISUAL ACUITY TEST

- Distance vision: Measures how well the patient can see at various distances using a Snellen chart or similar visual acuity chart. While presbyopia primarily affects near vision, it is important to assess overall visual acuity.

- Near vision: Assesses the patient's ability to see close-up text or objects. This is typically done using a near-vision chart with text of varying sizes.

REFRACTION TEST

- Subjective refraction: Determines the appropriate lens prescription needed to correct any refractive errors. The test involves using a phoropter or trial lenses to find the best correction for distance and near vision.

- Objective refraction: May include techniques such as retinoscopy, which helps to objectively measure the eye's refractive error.

ACCOMMODATION TESTING

- Push-up test: Measures the near point of accommodation (the closest point at which the patient can clearly see an object). The patient is asked to focus on a target that is moved closer until it becomes blurry.

- Minus lens test: Evaluates the eye's ability to focus on near objects by adding minus lenses and measuring how much additional power is required for clear vision.

BINOCULAR VISION ASSESSMENT

- Near point of convergence: Evaluates how well the eyes converge (turn inward) when focusing on a close object. Difficulty with convergence can be associated with presbyopia.

- Accommodation-convergence ratio: Assesses the relationship between accommodation (focusing) and convergence. A reduced ratio can indicate presbyopia.

PUPIL EXAMINATION

- Pupillary response: Evaluates the pupil's reaction to light and accommodation. While not directly diagnosing presbyopia, it helps rule out other conditions that affect visual function.

SLIT-LAMP EXAMINATION

- Anterior segment evaluation: A thorough examination of the anterior structures of the eye, including the cornea, lens and iris, to rule out other conditions such as cataracts that can affect vision.

FUNDOSCOPY

- Retinal examination: Using an ophthalmoscope, the retina and optic nerve are examined to rule out other underlying conditions, for example, diabetic retinopathy or macular degeneration.

DIAGNOSTIC IMAGING (IF NECESSARY)

- Ocular ultrasound or optical coherence tomography: In cases where additional evaluation is needed, imaging techniques including optical coherence tomography may be used to assess the condition of the retina and other structures.

PATIENT FEEDBACK

- Symptom correlation: Evaluating how well the patient's symptoms correlate with the findings from the tests. This helps in confirming the diagnosis and planning appropriate management.

In summary, the diagnosis of presbyopia involves a combination of visual acuity testing, refraction, accommodation assessment, binocular vision evaluation and sometimes additional imaging or examination to rule out other conditions. This comprehensive approach ensures an accurate diagnosis and helps in determining the most effective treatment options to manage presbyopia and improve the patient's quality of life.

MANAGEMENT

Without optical correction, presbyopia can significantly impact quality of life, causing issues with reading (such as difficulty with fine print, need for more lighting, diplopia, excessive tearing [epiphora], headaches, fatigue or eye strain [asthenopia]) and other activities that require seeing fine details up close, such as threading a needle (Katz et al. 2021).

The condition may be managed by optometrists (specialists in the diagnosis and management of refractive errors), orthoptists (specialists in ocular motility problems and assessment of refractive errors) or ophthalmologists (medically qualified physicians or surgeons).

Each eye is assessed individually for both near and distance vision. It is important that patients use their regular distance glasses or contact lenses during the test to identify any deterioration beyond their current prescription. Repeat the assessment using a pinhole occluder (see Chapter 2); if vision improves with the pinhole, it may indicate the presence of an uncorrected refractive error.

Managing presbyopia involves a range of strategies to help individuals with age-related loss of near vision maintain their daily functions and quality of life. The approach usually includes corrective lenses, lifestyle adjustments and, in some cases, surgical options (see Table 8.3).

HEALTH TEACHING

Presbyopia is a natural part of the ageing process of the eye. It is not a disease, and it cannot be prevented.

For individuals with presbyopia, effective health teaching is key to help them manage their condition and maintain their quality of life. Understanding the nature of presbyopia is the first step. It is important to explain that presbyopia is a natural part of ageing, where the eye's lens loses flexibility, making it difficult to focus on near objects. Symptoms such as difficulty reading small print, needing to hold reading materials at arm's length and experiencing eye strain or headaches should be addressed.

Information about corrective lenses is essential. Patients should be informed about the various options available, such as reading glasses, bifocals, trifocals and progressive lenses.

Table 8.3 The management of presbyopia

Management approach	Discussion
Corrective lenses	Reading glasses:
	Single vision lenses: These are the most common and are used specifically for near tasks. They are typically prescribed when individuals only need help with close-up work.
	Bifocals: These lenses have two distinct optical powers – one for distance and one for near vision. They are useful for people who need to switch between tasks at different distances.
	Trifocals: These lenses provide three different viewing zones: for distance, intermediate and near vision. They are suitable for people who need correction for all three types of vision.
	Progressive addition lenses (PALs): These provide a gradual change in lens power from the top (for distance vision) to the bottom (for near vision) without visible lines. PALs are often preferred for their aesthetic appeal and ease of use.
	Contact lenses:
	Multifocal contact lenses: These lenses have multiple zones of varying power to provide clear vision at different distances.
	Bifocal contact lenses: Designed with two distinct zones for near and distance vision.
	Monovision contact lenses: One eye is corrected for distance vision and the other for near vision.
Lifestyle adjustments	Lighting and visual aids:
	Enhanced lighting: Using brighter, more focused lighting can help reduce the strain on the eyes during close-up tasks.
	Magnifiers: Handheld or stand magnifiers can assist with reading small print.
Surgical options	Refractive surgery:
	Laser-assisted in situ keratomileusis (LASIK): Can be used to correct presbyopia by reshaping the cornea, though it is more commonly used for other refractive errors.
	Laser blended vision: A specific LASIK technique that creates a blend of distance and near-vision correction.
	Lens implants:
	Intraocular lenses: Multifocal or accommodating intraocular lenses can be implanted to replace the eye's natural lens, providing improved near and distance vision.
	Accommodating lenses: These lenses can shift position within the eye to focus at different distances.
Pharmacological treatments	Pharmaceutical interventions:
	Eye drops: Some new treatments involve eye drops that temporarily improve near vision by affecting the eye's accommodation.

Source: National Eye Institute (2019), Katz et al. (2021) and Moorfields Eye Hospital (2024).

Each type of lens has its own benefits and drawbacks and choosing the right one depends on individual needs. Patients should also be guided on how to use these lenses effectively and the importance of adhering to the prescribed lens power.

For those who prefer contact lenses, it is important to discuss options such as multifocal and bifocal contacts. Patients should be informed about how these lenses work and the benefits they provide. Additionally, proper care and maintenance of contact lenses should be emphasised to prevent infections and ensure optimal vision.

Lifestyle adjustments can significantly impact the management of presbyopia. Patients should be advised to use brighter and more focused lighting for tasks such as reading to reduce eye strain. Magnifying devices can be useful for reading small print or other close-up tasks, and adjustments to screen settings on computers and mobile devices, such as increasing text size and contrast, can also help.

In cases where patients are considering surgical options, such as LASIK, multifocal intraocular lenses or accommodating lenses, they should be provided with comprehensive information about these procedures. This includes discussing the potential benefits and risks, as well as pre- and post-surgical care to ensure optimal outcomes.

Ongoing eye care is vital. Patients should be encouraged to have regular eye tests to monitor changes in vision and update prescriptions as necessary. They should also be informed about symptoms that warrant immediate professional attention, such as sudden changes in vision or persistent discomfort.

Acknowledging the psychological and social impacts of vision changes is important. Patients may need support in adapting to these changes and suggesting support groups or online communities can provide them with a space to share experiences and strategies with others facing similar challenges.

By providing clear, practical information and support across these areas, those who offer care and support to people with presbyopia manage their condition effectively and enhance their quality of life.

CONCLUSION

Presbyopia is an inevitable aspect of the ageing process that affects nearly everyone to some degree, impacting their ability to see up close as they age. Understanding and managing this condition involves a multifaceted approach, tailored to meet the individual needs of each patient.

The diagnosis and management of presbyopia require a thorough understanding of its clinical presentation and the available corrective options. From simple reading glasses to advanced multifocal contact lenses and progressive lenses, a range of solutions are available to address the loss of near vision. For those seeking permanent solutions, surgical interventions such as LASIK or lens implants offer promising alternatives.

Lifestyle modifications, including the use of enhanced lighting and visual aids, can significantly improve daily functioning and quality of life. Regular eye examinations are essential to monitor changes and adjust prescriptions, ensuring that patients continue to benefit from the most appropriate corrective measures.

Providing people with information about presbyopia, its management strategies and available treatment options is key for empowering them to make informed decisions and adapt to changes in their vision. Addressing both the practical and emotional aspects of living with presbyopia helps in mitigating its impact on daily life.

As the population ages and the prevalence of presbyopia increases, ongoing research and advances in treatment options will continue to enhance our ability to manage this condition effectively. By combining clinical expertise with compassionate patient care, individuals can be helped to navigate the challenges of presbyopia and maintain their visual independence and overall quality of life.

GLOSSARY OF TERMS

Accommodation: The eye's ability to adjust focus for near and distance vision by changing the shape of the lens. With age, accommodation decreases, leading to presbyopia.

Astigmatism: A common vision condition caused by an irregular shape of the cornea or lens, leading to blurred or distorted vision. It can be present alongside presbyopia.

Bifocals: Eyeglasses with two distinct optical powers: one for distance vision and one for near vision. Used to correct presbyopia and other refractive errors.

Cataract: A clouding of the eye's natural lens, which can cause blurry vision. While distinct from presbyopia, cataract surgery can sometimes temporarily improve near vision.

Contact lenses: Lenses worn directly on the eye's surface to correct vision. Multifocal and bifocal contact lenses are designed to address presbyopia.

Distance vision: The ability to see objects clearly at a distance. Presbyopia primarily affects near vision, but maintaining good distance vision is also important.

Eye strain: Discomfort or fatigue in the eyes, often experienced with presbyopia when performing close-up tasks or after extended reading.

Intraocular lenses: Lenses implanted in the eye during cataract surgery or as a refractive procedure. Multifocal or accommodating intraocular lenses can address presbyopia.

Laser-assisted in situ keratomileusis (LASIK): A type of refractive eye surgery that reshapes the cornea to improve vision. It is not typically used to treat presbyopia but may be combined with other procedures.

Multifocal lenses: Lenses that provide multiple focal points for clear vision at various distances, commonly used in glasses and contact lenses to manage presbyopia.

Optical coherence tomography: A non-invasive imaging technique used to capture high-resolution images of the retina and other eye structures, helpful in assessing overall eye health and related conditions.

Pinhole test: A diagnostic test where the patient looks through a small pinhole to determine if vision improves, which can indicate an uncorrected refractive error.

Progressive addition lenses: Eyeglasses that offer a gradual change in lens power from top to bottom, providing a seamless transition from distance to near vision without visible lines.

Presbyopia: An age-related condition where the eye's lens loses flexibility, making it difficult to focus on near objects. It typically begins in the early to mid-40s.

Refractive error: A general term for vision problems caused by the eye's inability to properly focus light, including conditions such as myopia, hyperopia, astigmatism and presbyopia.

Trifocals: Eyeglasses with three distinct optical powers for distance, intermediate and near vision. They are designed to help individuals with presbyopia and other visual needs.

Visual acuity: The clarity or sharpness of vision, often measured using an eye chart. Presbyopia typically affects near visual acuity.

MULTIPLE CHOICE QUESTIONS

1. What is presbyopia?
   a) A condition where the eye's lens becomes too flexible
   b) A type of cataract
   c) An age-related loss of near vision due to decreased lens flexibility
   d) A refractive error caused by an irregular cornea

2. At what age does presbyopia typically begin?
   a) 20–30 years
   b) 30–40 years
   c) 40–50 years
   d) 50–60 years

3. Which of the following is a common symptom of presbyopia?
   a) Difficulty seeing objects at a distance
   b) Double vision
   c) Blurred vision up close
   d) Sudden loss of vision

4. What does the pinhole test help determine in the context of presbyopia?
   a) The presence of cataracts
   b) Improvement in vision due to uncorrected refractive error
   c) The presence of macular degeneration
   d) The need for eye surgery

5. Which surgical option is commonly used to manage presbyopia?
   a) Laser-assisted in situ keratomileusis (LASIK)
   b) Cataract surgery
   c) Refractive lens exchange
   d) Glaucoma surgery

6. What does the term 'accommodating lenses' refer to?
   a) Lenses that change power based on distance
   b) Lenses that have multiple fixed focal points
   c) Lenses that only correct for distance
   d) Lenses that are used for near vision only

7. What is the main cause of presbyopia?
    a) Irregular corneal shape
    b) Loss of lens elasticity
    c) High blood pressure
    d) Increased intraocular pressure

8. What is the typical impact of presbyopia on reading?
    a) Improved reading speed
    b) Difficulty reading small print
    c) Increased ability to read in low light
    d) No impact on reading ability

9. Which of the following conditions is often mistaken for presbyopia?
    a) Myopia
    b) Astigmatism
    c) Cataracts
    d) Glaucoma

10. What type of lighting is recommended to alleviate symptoms of presbyopia?
    a) Dim and indirect lighting
    b) Bright and focused lighting
    c) Fluorescent lighting
    d) Natural sunlight

REFERENCES

Borooah, S. and Tint, N.L. (2023). The visual system (Chapter 8). In: *Macleod's Clinical Examination*, 15e (eds. A.R. Dover, J.A. Innes, and K. Fairhurst). London: Elsevier.

Castagno, V.D., Fassa, A.G., Carret, M.L. et al. (2014). Hyperopia: a meta-analysis of prevalence and a review of associated factors among school-aged children. *BMC Ophthalmology* 14: 163. doi: 10.1186/1471-2415-14-163.

Clare, C. (2020). The senses (Chapter 15). In: *Fundamentals of Anatomy and Physiology*, 3e (eds. I. Peate and S. Evans). Oxford: Wiley.

Cochrane, G.M., du Toit, R., and Le Mesurier, R.T. (2010). Management of refractive errors. *British Medical Journal* 340: c1711. doi: 10.1136/bmj.c1711.

Cooper, J. and Tkatchenko, A.V. (2018). A review of current concepts of the etiology and treatment of myopia. *Eye Contact Lens* 44 (4): 231–247. doi: 10.1097/ICL.000000000000499.

Galloway, N.R., Amoaku, W.M.K., Galloway, P.H., et al. (2023). *Common Eye Diseases and their Management*. Springer Nature. doi: 10.1007/978-3-031-08450-8_23.

Hagler, D., Harding, M.M., Kwong, J. et al. (2023). *Lewis's Medical-Surgical Nursing*. St Louis: Elsevier.

Huether, S.E. and Rodway, G.W. (2019). Pain, temperature regulation, sleep, and sensory function (Chapter 16). In: *Pathophysiology. The Biologic Basis for Disease in Adults and Children*, 8e (eds. K.L. McCance and S.E. Huether). St Louis: Elsevier.

Jarvis, C. and Eckhardt, A. (2024). *Physical Examination and Health Assessment*, 9e. St Louis: Elsevier.

Katz, J.A., Karpecki, P.M., Dorca, A. et al. (2021). Presbyopia—a review of current treatment options and emerging therapies. *Clinical Ophthalmology* 24 (15): 2167–2178. doi: 10.2147/OPTH.S259011.

Little, J.A., Congdon, N.G., Resnikoff, S. et al. (2024). Global estimates on the number of people blind or visually impaired by uncorrected refractive error: a meta-analysis from 2000 to 2020. *Eye* 38 (11): 2083–2101. doi: 10.1038/s41433-024-03106-0.

Moorfields Eye Hospital (2024). Presbyopia. https://www.moorfields.nhs.uk/eye-conditions/presbyopia (accessed August 2024).

National Eye Institute (2019). Eyeglasses for refractive errors. https://www.nei.nih.gov/learn-about-eye-health/eye-conditions-and-diseases/refractive-errors/eyeglasses-refractive-errors (accessed August 2024).

Needham, Y. (2019). Ophthalmological disorders (Chapter 38). In: *Learning to Care* (ed. I. Peate). London: Elsevier.

Royal National Institute of Blind People (2021). Key statistics about sight loss. https://media.rnib.org.uk/documents/Key_stats_about_sight_loss_2021.pdf (accessed August 2024).

Torricelli, A.A., Junior, J.B., Santhiago, M.R. et al. (2012). Surgical management of presbyopia. *Clinical Ophthalmology* 6: 1459–1466. doi: 10.2147/OPTH.S35533.

Wang, L.L., Wang, W., Han, X.T. et al. (2018). Influence of severity and types of astigmatism on visual acuity in school-aged children in southern China. *International Journal of Ophthalmology* 11 (8): 1377–1383. doi: 10.18240/ijo.2018.08.20.

World Health Organization (2019). World vision report. https://iris.who.int/bitstream/handle/10665/328717/9789241516570-eng.pdf?sequence=18 (accessed August 2024).

MCQ Answers

Chapter 1   Anatomy and Physiology: The Eyes

1. (b); 2. (b); 3. (d); 4. (b); 5. (c); 6. (b); 7. (b); 8. (b); 9. (b); 10. (b).

Chapter 2   Assessment of the Eyes

1. (d); 2. (b); 3. (b); 4. (a); 5. (b); 6. (b); 7. (b); 8. (b); 9. (b); 10. (b).

Chapter 3   Glaucoma

1. (c); 2. (c); 3. (b); 4. (b); 5. (c); 6. (b); 7. (b); 8. (b); 9. (c); 10. (c).

Chapter 4   Cataract

1. (b); 2. (c); 3. (c); 4. (b); 5. (c); 6. (c); 7. (b); 8. (c); 9. (c); 10. (c).

Chapter 5   Conjunctivitis

1. (c); 2. (c); 3. (c); 4. (c); 5. (c); 6. (c); 7. (c); 8. (b); 9. (b); 10. (b).

Chapter 6   Age-related Macular Degeneration

1. (b); 2. (b); 3. (c); 4. (c); 5. (b); 6. (c); 7. (c); 8. (a); 9. (a); 10. (b).

Chapter 7   Retinitis

1. (b); 2. (b); 3. (b); 4. (b); 5. (a); 6. (d); 7. (b); 8. (c); 9. (b); 10. (c).

Chapter 8   Presbyopia

1. (c); 2. (c); 3. (c); 4. (b); 5. (c); 6. (a); 7. (b); 8. (b); 9. (c); 10. (b).

Index

Note: Page numbers in *italics* and **bold** refers to figures and tables respectively.

A

accommodating intra-optical
  lenses, 66
accommodating lenses, 144
accommodation, 136
  changes with age and, 136–137
  importance of, 137
  mechanism of, 136
  reflex, 136
  testing for presbyopia, 142
accommodation-convergence
  ratio, 142
adaptive strategies, 127
adeno-associated virus vector, 128
age factors for presbyopia, 139
age-related macular degeneration
  (AMD), 63, 94, 138
  Amsler grid test, 106
  clinical investigations and
    diagnosis, 103
  clinical presentation, 100
  documentation and
    follow-up, 105–106
  dry AMD, 95–97, 101
  electroretinography, 107
  epidemiology, 99
  fluorescein angiography, 107
  fundoscopic examination, 106
  fundus autofluorescence, 107
  general symptoms of, 102–103
  health teaching, 109–110
  indocyanine green
    angiography, 107
  initial consultation, 103–104
  macular degeneration, 94–95
  management, 107–108
  optical coherence
    tomography, 106
  pathophysiological changes
    associated with, 95
  risk factors, 99–100, 100
  structured interviews and
    questionnaires, 104
  symptom inquiry, 104
  visual acuity test, 106
  wet AMD, 97–99, 101–102

allergic conjunctivitis, 73, 76
  clinical features
    associated with, 82
  medications, 88
  risk factors of, 79
alpha agonists, 46
amblyopia, 22, 63
American Academy of
  Ophthalmology, 95
Amsler grid test, 32, 104, 106
angle-closure glaucoma, 38, 39, 47
anterior segment evaluation, 142
antihistamine eye drops, 88
antioxidants, 57
anti-VEGF therapy, 108
aqueous humour, 39
aqueous veins, 39
argon laser trabeculoplasty, 45
artificial intraocular lens, 59
artificial lens, 65
artificial tears, 73, 88, 89
A-scan ultrasound biometry, 64
assistive technology, 127
asthenopia, 143
astigmatism, 21, 135
atrophic AMD, 95
attenuation of retinal blood
  vessels, 117
autosomal dominant, 115, 118
autosomal recessive, 115, 118
axial length, 65

B

bacterial conjunctivitis, 73,
  76, 87. *see also* viral
  conjunctivitis
  clinical features
    associated with, 81
  hygiene measures, 87–88
  risk factors of, 79
  topical antibiotics, 87
Best disease. *see* genetic disorder
beta blockers, 46
bifocal, 143, 144
  contact lenses, 144, 145
binocular diplopia, 60

binocular vision, 22
  assessment, 142
  testing, 30
biomicroscopy. *see* slit-lamp
  examination
bioptic telescopes, 127
blepharitis, 6, 77
blind spot, 30
blurred vision, 60
bone spicules, 121, 125
bulbar conjunctiva, 6

C

canthus
  lateral commissure, 5–6
  medial commissure, 6–7
capsule, 70
carbonic anhydrase inhibitors, 46
cartella, 66
cataract, 54–55, 138, 140, 142
  clinical investigations and
    diagnosis, 61
  clinical presentation, 59–61
  environmental and lifestyle
    factors, 58
  epidemiology, 58–59
  examination and
    investigations, 63, 63–64
  genetic and molecular
    factors, 58
  health teaching, 66, 66–69
  intra-optical lenses, types of, 66
  lens fibre cell changes, 58
  management, 64–65
  normal lens and lens affected
    by cataract, 54
  oxidative stress and free radical
    damage, 57
  pathophysiological changes
    associated with, 56
  patient history, 61–62
  postoperative care, 66
  protein aggregation and
    crystallin changes, 57
  risk factors associated
    with, 56–57, 59

cataract (*Cont.*)
   surgery, 3, 25, 65
   surgical management, 65
   systemic diseases and
      medications, 58
   types of, 55
   water and ion imbalance, 58
Caucasian ethnicity, 99
cell differentiation, 58
cellular damage and repair, 76
central serous
      chorioretinopathy, 94
central vision
   changes, 123
   loss, 115, 121
chaperone, provision of, 105
chemical conjunctivitis, 73–74, 77
   management, 88–89
   risk factors of, 79
chemosis, 75
chorioretinal atrophy, 96
choroidal neovascularisation, 94,
      97–98, 101
choroideraemia, 114
chronic conjunctivitis, 82
chronic dacryocystitis, 78
chronic low-grade
      inflammation, 97
chronic vision loss, 124
ciliary body, 45
ciliary epithelium, 39
ciliary muscle
   contraction, 136
   relaxation, 136
   weakening, 137
closed-angle glaucoma. *see*
      angle-closure glaucoma
colour blindness, 22, 30
colour vision, 10–11, 22
   assessment, 30
   deficiency, 115, 121
   testing, 21
combination drugs, 46
commissure, 5
comprehensive care
   coordination approach, 3
   planning, 21
comprehensive eye examination
   for cataracts, 63
comprehensive past medical
      history, 25
comprehensive vision
      assessment, 21
cone photoreceptors, 116
cone–rod dystrophy, 114
confrontation test, 30
congenital cataracts, 55
congenital glaucoma, 38

conjunctiva, 6, 74
conjunctival redness, 85
conjunctivitis, 73
   allergic, 73, 76
   bacterial, 73, 76
   cellular damage and repair, 76
   chemical, 73–74, 77
   clinical examination, 85–86
   clinical investigations and
      diagnosis, 83
   clinical presentation, 81, 81–82
   conjunctival anatomy and
      function, 75
   epidemiology, 78
   eye and associated
      structures, 75
   general risks, 80
   giant papillary, 74, 77
   health teaching, 89, 89–90
   immune cell infiltration, 76
   increased vascular
      permeability, 75
   investigations, 86–87, 86–87
   management, 87–89
   mucous and tear production, 76
   neonatal, 74, 77
   non-infectious, 74, 77
   ophthalmia neonatorum, 78–79
   pathophysiological changes
      associated with, 74
   patient history, 83–85
   populations at higher
      risk, 80–81
   protective mechanisms and
      self-limiting
      nature, 77–78
   Report, Remove, Rinse
      guidance, 83
   risk factors, 79, 79
   types and specific
      pathophysiological
      mechanisms, 76
   vasodilation and increased
      blood flow, 75
   viral, 73, 76
contact lens, 144
   use of, 84
   wearers, 80
contrast sensitivity test for
      cataracts, 63
corneal curvature, 65
corneal thickness assessment, 44
corneal topography, 32
corrective lenses, 143, 144
cortical cataracts, 55
corticosteroids, 41, 91
cromolyn sodium, 91
crystallin changes, 57

cupping of optic disc, 42
cup-to-disc ratio, 42
cyclophotocoagulation, 45

D
dacryocystitis, 6
dark adaptation test, 126
debris
   barrier against moisture and, 4
   protection, 5
degenerated macula, *96*
depth perception, 21
diabetes, cataract and, 58
diabetic retinopathy, 3, 20, 63, 138
diagnostic tests, in
      ophthalmology, 31–33
diplopia
   binocular, 60
   monocular, 60
direct ophthalmoscopy, 34
discharge, 74, 75, 81, 83
disciform scar formation, 98
distance vision, 28, 142
diurnal variation, 50
double vision in one eye, 60
Driving Vehicle and Licencing
      Agency, 48
drusen formation, 96
dry age-related macular
      degeneration, 95, 108. *see*
      also wet age-related
      macular degeneration
   absence of key features in, 97
   advanced stages, 101
   chorioretinal atrophy, 96
   differences between wet AMD
      and, 102–103
   drusen formation, 96
   early stages, 101
   inflammatory and oxidative
      stress, 97
   intermediate stages, 101
   retinal pigment epithelium
      changes, 96

E
early-onset retinitis pigmentosa,
      120, 121–122
ectropion, 77
educational barriers, 3
electrodiagnostic testing, 32
electronic magnifiers, 127
electroretinogram, 121
electroretinography, 32, 107, 126
elevated IOP, 39, 41
emmetropia, 134
emotional impact of glaucoma, 48
enhanced lighting, 144

environmental factors for
  presbyopia, 139
epiphora, 6, 143
exfoliative glaucoma, 38
external examination, 34
exudative AMD, 97
eye, 8, *54*
  accessory structures of, *4*
  anatomy and physiology of, 4–7
  anatomy in
    accommodation, 136
  assessment of, 21–23
  central processing of visual
    information, 15–16
  chambers, 12
  clinical findings from eye
    examination, 23
  colour vision assessment, 30
  diagnostic tests, 31, 31–33
  documentation of
    findings, 24–27
  drops, 144
  fibrous tunic, 9
  focal length, 13–14
  health examination, 22
  hyperopia, 14
  lacrimal apparatus, 7–8
  LogMAR vision testing, 29
  myopia, 14
  neural tunic, 10
  patient history in ophthalmic
    assessment, 24
  presbyopia, 14
  processing of visual
    information, 15
  refraction, 12–13
  sense of sight, 1–4
  showing position of macula, *95*
  strain, 141, 143, 145
  surgery for presbyopia, 140
  testing visual function, 27–29
  tumbling 'E', 'E' test, 29–30
  vascular tunic, 9
  vision assessment, 20–21
eyebrows, 4–5
eyelashes, 5
eyelids, 5
  examination, 85

F

fading of colours, cataracts and, 60
family history
  for retinal dystrophies, 123
  for retinitis
    pigmentosa, 118, 118
  for vision assessment, 25
farsightedness, 135
fibre cell integrity, 58

fibrous tunic, 9
fluid accumulation, 101
fluorescein angiography, 31, 107
focal length, 13–14
follicles, 81
free radical damage, 57
functional history, eyes
    assessment and, 26
functional tests, 126
fundoscopic examination, 106
fundoscopy, 142
fundus autofluorescence, 107, 126
fundus photography, 32, 121, 125

G

gender factors for presbyopia, 140
gene therapy, 128
genetic counselling, 118
genetic counsellor, 118
genetic disorder, 94
genetic mutations, 116, 118
  family history, 118
  genetic variability, 119
  inherited mutations, 118–119
  phenotypic variability, 119
genetic predisposition, 62, 139
genetic screening, 126
genetic testing, 126
genetic variability, 119
geographic atrophy. *see*
    chorioretinal atrophy
giant papillary
    conjunctivitis, 74, 77
glare, sensitivity to, 60, 61
glare testing for cataracts, 64
glaucoma, 3, 20, 37, 40, 63, 138
  approaches to
    management of, 45–46
  clinical investigations and
    diagnosis, 43
  clinical presentation, 42–43
  discussions regarding risk
    factors, 43
  drainage devices, 46
  emergency situations, 48–49
  epidemiology, 39–40
  examination and
    investigations, 44
  family history, 43
  lifestyle and environmental
    factors, 44
  management, 44–48
  pathophysiological changes
    associated with, 37–39
  patient history, 43
  risk factors, 41, 41–42
  types of, 38
glial cell activation, 117

gonioscopy, 33, 44

H

Haemophilus influenzae, 73
haemorrhage, 98
halos around lights, 60
handheld magnifiers, 127
health conditions, for
    presbyopia, 139
health teaching
  for age-related macular
    degeneration, 109–110
  for cataract, 66, 66–69
  for glaucoma, 47
  for people with age-related
    macular
    degeneration, 109–110
  for presbyopia, 143–145
  for retinal dystrophies, 129
  for retinitis
    pigmentosa, 129, 129
herpes simplex virus, 78
histamine, 76
history taking, for cataract, 62
human communication, 1
hyperaemia, 75
hyperopia, 14, 21, 134

I

IgE blood tests, 87
immune cell infiltration, 76
immunocompromised
    individuals, 80
incisional surgery, 45, 46, 47
indirect ophthalmoscopy, 34
indocyanine green
    angiography, 107
infectious conjunctivitis, 78
inflammation
  dry AMD and, 97
  response, 97, 117
  wet AMD and, 98, 98
information processing, 1
informed consent, 106
inheritance patterns, 118
inherited mutations, 118–119
inherited retinal
    degenerations, 114
intraocular lens (IOL), 59,
    144, 145
intraocular pressure (IOP), 31,
    34, 37, 39
  maintaining, 37
  raised, 37, 42
intra-optical lenses, types of, 66
IOL. *see* intraocular lens (IOL)
IOP. *see* intraocular pressure (IOP)
Ishihara plates, 30

J

juvenile glaucoma, 38
juvenile macular degeneration, 94

L

lacrimal apparatus, 7–8, *7*
lacrimal caruncle, 5
lacrimal gland, 7
laser-assisted in situ keratomileusis
    (LASIK), 25, 62, 140, 144
laser blended vision, 144
laser peripheral iridotomy, 45
laser surgery, 45, *45*, 47
LASIK. *see* laser-assisted in situ
    keratomileusis (LASIK)
late-onset retinitis
    pigmentosa, 120, 122
lateral commissure, 5–6
Leber congenital amaurosis, 114
lens, 54, *54*, 55, 56, 57
    implants, 144
lifestyle factors
    adjustments for presbyopia, 144
    for cataract, 58
    for glaucoma, 44
    for presbyopia, 140
    retinal dystrophies, 119
    for vision assessment, 26
lighting aids, 144
local anaesthesia, 65
localised macular oedema, 98
LogMAR vision testing, 29
loss of central vision, 121
low-tension glaucoma. *see*
    normal-tension glaucoma
low vision aids, 108, 109, 110
lymphadenopathy, 84, 86

M

macula, 31, 34, 116
    degenerated, *96*
    eye showing position of, *95*
    normal, *96*
macular degeneration, 3, 20,
    22, 25, 29
    secondary to other
        conditions, 94
magnifiers, 144
    electronic, 127
    handheld, 127
mast cell stabilisers, 88
medial commissure, 6–7
medications, 45, 46
    approaches to improving
        concordance, 48–49
    for presbyopia, 139
Meibomian gland
    dysfunction, 82

metamorphopsia, 101, 104
microglial activation, 117
minimally invasive glaucoma
    surgery, 46
minus lens test, 142
monocular diplopia, 60
monofocal intra-optical lenses, 66
monovision contact lenses, 144
mucous and tear production, 76
multidisciplinary approach, 21
multifocal contact lenses, 144, 145
multifocal intra-optical lenses, 66
myopia, 14, 21, 134
myopic macular degeneration, 94

N

narrow-angle glaucoma. *see*
    angle-closure glaucoma
National Institute for Health and
    Care Excellence (NICE), 37
near point of convergence, 142
near-sightedness, 135
near-vision testing, 29, 142
neonatal conjunctivitis, 74, 77
neonates, 80
neovascular AMD, 97
neovascular glaucoma, 38
neural tunic, 10
NICE. *see* National Institute for
    Health and Care
    Excellence (NICE)
night blindness, 115, 120, 122
night vision, difficulty with, 60
non-exudative AMD, 95
non-infectious
    conjunctivitis, 74, 77
    clinical features
        associated with, 82
normal macula, *96*
normal-pressure glaucoma. *see*
    normal-tension glaucoma
normal-tension glaucoma, 38
nuclear cataracts, 55
nyctalopia. *see* night blindness

O

objective refraction, 142
occupational hazards, 62
occupational history, eyes
    assessment and, 25–26
occupation factors for
    presbyopia, 139
OCT. *see* optical coherence
    tomography (OCT)
ocular diseases, 25
ocular ultrasound, 143
open-angle glaucoma, 39
ophthalmia neonatorum, 78–79, 80

ophthalmic assessment, patient
    history in, 24
ophthalmologists, 143
ophthalmology, diagnostic
    tests in, 31–33
ophthalmoscopy, 31, 106
optical aids, 127
optical coherence tomography
    (OCT), 31, 64, 106,
    121, 125, 143
    angiography, 126
optic disc, 31, 34
    cupping of, 42
    examination, 44
optic nerve, 37, 39, 42
optic nerve atrophy, 39, 117
optometrists, 143
orthoptists, 143
oxidative damage, 97
oxidative stress, 57, 97
    dry AMD and, 97
    reducing, 119
    wet AMD and, 98

P

pachymetry, 32
palpebrae. *see* eyelids
palpebral conjunctiva, 6
PALs. *see* progressive addition
    lenses (PALs)
papillae, 77
patchy vision loss, 39
patient-centred care plans, 3
patient education, 89, 108
patient feedback for
    presbyopia, 143
patient history
    for cataract, 61–62
    for conjunctivitis, 83–85
    for glaucoma, 43
    in ophthalmic assessment, 24
    for presbyopia, 141
    for retinal dystrophies, 122
PCO. *see* posterior capsule
    opacification (PCO)
perimeter, 30
perimetry, 44, 127
peripheral vision, 21
    loss, 42, 48, 115, 120, 123
phacoemulsification, 65, *65*
phenotypic variability, 119
photodynamic therapy, 108, 110
photophobia, 24, 60, 115, 121
photoreceptor degeneration, 116
photoreceptors, 116
photorefractive
    keratectomy (PRK), 62
pigmentary glaucoma, 38

pigment epithelium
    detachment, 111
pigment migration, 117
pigmentosa, 116
pinhole test, 143
pink eye. *see* conjunctivitis
polymerase chain reaction
    testing, 86
posterior capsule
    opacification (PCO), 66
posterior subcapsular cataracts, 55
postoperative care, 66
postoperative eye cleansing, 66
preauricular lymph nodes, 86
presbyopia, 14, 134, 135
    clinical investigations and
        diagnosis, 140
    clinical presentation, 140
    epidemiology, 137
    health teaching, 143–145
    management, 143, 144
    pathophysiological
        changes associated
        with, 134–137
    risk factors, 138–140
    signs and symptoms
        associated with, 141
primary open-angle glaucoma,
    47, 37, 38
    pathophysiological changes
        associated with, 37–39
    symptoms of, 42
prism glasses, 127
PRK. *see* photorefractive
    keratectomy (PRK)
progressive addition lenses
    (PALs), 144
progressive vision loss, 120–121
prostaglandins, 46
protective mechanisms of
    conjunctivitis, 77
protein aggregation, 57
pseudomembranes, 86
ptosis, 27
public health education, 3
pupil
    examination, 23, 142
    presbyopia and, 137
    size and reactivity, assessing, 28
pupillary constriction, 136
purulent discharge, 76, 81, 85
push-up test, 142

R

radiation cataracts, 55
reactive oxygen species (ROS),
    57, 69, 97

reading difficulty, cataracts and, 61
reading glasses, 144
redness, *23*
refraction, 12–13
    test for presbyopia, 142
refractive correction, 64
refractive error, 134, 137
    for presbyopia, 139
refractive surgery, 144
refractory disorders, 135
retina, 10, 21, 22
    architecture of, 117
    cross-section of, *11*
    focal length, 13–14
    focusing images on, 12
    organisation of, 10
    photoreceptors, 116
    rods and cones, *12*
    structure, colour vision
        and, 10–11
retinal changes, 121
retinal detachment, 25, 30
retinal dystrophies, 114
    additional tests, 126
    age of onset, 120
    causes, 115
    central vision changes, 123
    clinical examination, 125
    clinical implications, 117–118
    clinical investigations and
        diagnosis, 122
    clinical presentation, 120
    environmental and lifestyle
        factors, 119
    epidemiology, 118
    examination and
        investigations, 125
    family history, 123
    functional tests, 126
    gene therapy, 128
    genetic mutations, 116
    genetic mutations, 118–119
    genetic testing, 126
    health teaching, 129
    inflammatory responses, 117
    initial symptoms, 120–122
    management, 127–128
    pathophysiological changes
        associated with, 116
    patient history, 122
    photoreceptor
        degeneration, 116
    previous ocular and medical
        history, 123–124
    psychosocial aspects,
        124–125
    retinal imaging, 125–126

retinal pigment epithelium
    changes, 117
retinal remodelling, 117
    risk factors, 118
    secondary effects, 117
    symptom onset and
        progression, 122–123
    symptoms, 115
    types, 114
    vascular changes, 117
    visual field testing, 127
    visual function impact, 124
retinal examination
    for cataracts, 63
    for presbyopia, 142
retinal imaging, 125–126
retinal layers, *115*
retinal pigment epithelial
    detachment, 98
retinal pigment
    epithelium (RPE), 94
    changes, 96, 117
    dysfunction, 117
retinal remodelling, 117
retinitis, 116
retinitis pigmentosa, 114, 116
rod photoreceptors, 116
ROS. *see* reactive oxygen
    species (ROS)
Royal College of
    Ophthalmologists, 95
Royal National Institute of Blind
    People, 22, 127, 138
RPE. *see* retinal pigment
    epithelium (RPE)
RPE65 gene, 128

S

Schirmer test, 87
Schlemm's canal, 39
scotoma, 101, 104
sebaceous glands, 5
secondary cataracts, 55
secondary glaucoma, 38
selective laser
    trabeculoplasty (SLT), 45
self-limiting nature of
    conjunctivitis, 77
senses, 4
sensory organs, 4
sight
    loss, 138
    sense of, 1–4, 2
single vision lenses, 144
skin prick tests, 87
slit-lamp examination
    for cataracts, 63

slit-lamp examination (*Cont.*)
of conjunctivitis, 86
for presbyopia, 142
for vision assessment, 27, 31
SLT. *see* selective laser
trabeculoplasty (SLT)
Snellen test-type charts, 28, *28*
social history, eyes assessment
and, 25–26
sorbitol, 58
specular microscopy, 33, 64
Staphylococcus aureus, 73
Stargardt disease, 114. *see also*
juvenile macular
degeneration
steroids, 67
strabismus, 22
Streptococcus pneumonia, 73
structured interviews and
questionnaires, 104
subjective refraction, 142
submandibular lymph nodes, 86
submaxillary lymph nodes. *see*
submandibular
lymph nodes
subretinal haemorrhage, 101
subretinal injection, 131
supportive care, 108
sweat glands, 5
systemic diseases, 25
and medications for cataract, 58
systemic medical health, 25
systemic review, 26

T
TBUT. *see* tear break-up
time (TBUT)
tear break-up time (TBUT), 87
tear drainage disorders, 6
tear drainage system, 6
tear production, mucous and, 76
technological aids, 3
tonometry, 31, 64
optic disc examination, 44
topical antibiotics, 87
trabecular meshwork, 39
trabeculectomy, 46
traumatic cataracts, 55
trifocals, 143, 144
tumbling 'E', 'E' test, 29–30
tunnel vision, 115, 117, 120, 123

U
ultrafiltration, 39
ultrasound biomicroscopy, 32
ultraviolet (UV), 56, 57, 58
protection, 69, 69
uncorrected refractive error, 134
Usher syndrome, 127
UV. *see* ultraviolet (UV)
uvea, 9

V
vascular changes, 117
vascular occlusions, 25
vascular tunic, 9
vasodilation, 75
VFQ-25. *see* Visual Functioning
Questionnaire (VFQ-25)
viral conjunctivitis, 73, 76.
see also bacterial
conjunctivitis
antiviral medications, 88
clinical features
associated with, 81
hygiene measures, 88
risk factors of, 79
supportive care, 88
vision assessment, 20
comprehensive care
planning, 21
ensuring safe environment, 20
identifying potential risks, 20
preserving independence, 20
reporting changes in visual
acuity, 20–21
vision loss, 3
visual acuity, 21, 28, 43
reduced, 121
reporting changes in, 20–21
visual acuity test, 31
for age-related macular
degeneration, 106
for presbyopia, 142
for retinal dystrophies, 125
visual aids, 1, 144
visual field, 44
assessment, 30
loss, 42–43
test, 21, 42, 44, 127
visual function
impact, 124
testing, 27–29

visual functioning index, 104
Visual Functioning Questionnaire
(VFQ-25), 104
visual history, eyes
assessment and, 26
visual impairment, 2
statistics in UK, 138
visual information
central processing of, 15–16
processing of, 15
visual inspections, 1
visual perception, 1
visual stimuli, 20
Vitamin A, 116
vitelliform macular dystrophy, 114
voretigene neparvovec, 128

W
wet age-related macular
degeneration, 97, 108. *see
also* dry age-related
macular degeneration
advanced stages, 102
choroidal neovascularisation,
97–98
differences between dry AMD
and, 102–103
formation of disciform scar, 98
genetic and environmental
factors, 98–99
localised macular oedema and
haemorrhage, 98
oxidative stress and
inflammation, 98
retinal pigment epithelial
detachment, 98
sudden onset, 101
symptoms, 101–102
whole-exome sequencing or
targeted gene panels, 126

X
X-linked manner, 115, 119

Y
yellowing of colours,
cataracts and, 60
yttrium aluminium garnet laser
capsulotomy (YAG laser
capsulotomy), 55, 66